WHAT PEOPLE ARE SAYING ABOUT . . .

Wheat-Free Recipes & Menus:

Delicious, Healthful Eating for People with Food Sensitivities

by Carol Fenster, Ph.D.

"Carol Fenster, Ph.D., is a recognized expert regarding the gluten-free diet. Once again she has written an outstanding cookbook and guide for patients with celiac disease and dermatitis herpetiformis and for others who elect to follow the healthy, gluten-free lifestyle."

—CYNTHIA S. RUDERT, M.D., F.A.C.P.
Medical Adviser, Celiac Disease Foundation
Medical Adviser, Gluten Intolerance Group
Medical Director, Gluten Sensitive Support Group of Atlanta

"This is my favorite recipe book during our GIG Kid's Summer Camp. We have so many children with multiple food sensitivities, and this book makes it easy to find the perfect recipe."

—CYNTHIA KUPPER, R.D., C.D.
Executive Director, Gluten Intolerance Group

"Anyone who thinks the wheat-free diet is restrictive hasn't seen *Wheat-Free Recipes & Menus* yet. Loaded with unique and flavor-filled recipes, menu suggestions, and ideas for wheat substitutions, this book helps people focus on the vast and wonderful foods they *can* eat."

—DANNA KORN
Founder, R.O.C.K. (Raising Our Celiac Kids)

"Carol Fenster's calm, clear guidance inspires hope that everyone can cook 'normal' food prepared without gluten that is as delicious and nutritious as the wheat-containing food they are used to."

—ANN WHELAN
Editor/Publisher, Gluten-Free Living *magazine*

"If you are wheat- or gluten-sensitive, there's no need to feel deprived. Carol Fenster shows how to make excellent substitutes for all your favorites in terms of sample menus and recipes for breads, pasta, desserts, sauces, vegetables, poultry, fish, and meat dishes. Put more variety into your gluten-free, wheat-free diet with Carol!"

—JANET Y. RINEHART
Former President, CSA/USA, Inc.
Chairman, Houston Celiac Support Group

"Carol Fenster's cookbook is a compassionate guide for the newly diagnosed celiac, explaining the merits of flour blends and how to find hidden sources of gluten. A godsend for the 2.2 million Americans with celiac disease, these pages are a road map to the finest gluten-free comfort food around."

—MICHELLE MELIN-ROGOVIN, M.P.P.
Program Director, University of Chicago Celiac Disease Program

"An amazing compilation of fabulous recipes, menus, and ingredient resources for anyone trying to cook without wheat, gluten, or casein."

—MARTHA S. STEFFEN, P.A.-C.
Colorado Allergy and Asthma Centers, P.C.

Wheat-Free Recipes & Menus

Delicious, Healthful Eating for People with Food Sensitivities

REVISED AND EXPANDED

Carol Fenster, Ph.D.

AVERY ■ A MEMBER OF PENGUIN GROUP (USA) INC. ■ NEW YORK

a member of
Penguin Group (USA) Inc.
375 Hudson Street
New York, NY 10014
www.penguin.com

Library of Congress Cataloging-in-Publication Data

Fenster, Carol Lee.
Wheat-free recipes & menus: delicious, healthful eating for people with food sensitivities / Carol Fenster
p.   cm.
Includes index.
ISBN 1-58333-191-3
1. Wheat-free diet—Recipes.   2. Gluten-free diet—Recipes.   I. Title.
RM237.87.F463   2004   2003063745
641.5'637—dc22

Printed in the United States of America
7   9   10   8   6

Book design by Meighan Cavanaugh

Line art by Lisa Daly, GoodCompany

This book is dedicated to Larry, Brett, Helke, and Keene,
and to the memory of my mother, who first introduced me to cooking.

Acknowledgments

The idea for this book came from my own need for a life without gluten. So much has changed since it was originally published in 1995. Back then, my book was one of a mere handful of resources for the gluten-free lifestyle, and the medical profession still thought celiac disease was a rare condition. Today, research centers at major universities are focused on gluten intolerance; several national nonprofit associations offer dietary guidance; the American Dietetic Association has guidelines for the gluten-free diet; and the number of companies providing gluten-free products has grown from that mere handful in 1995 to more than a hundred, worldwide.

Along the way, from that original version in 1995 to this latest version, the book has been nurtured and supported by many people. I am thankful for the support of several experts in the medical and gluten-free community, including Cynthia S. Rudert, M.D., Cynthia Kupper, R.D., C.D., Martha S. Steffen, P.A.-C., Michelle Melin-Rogovin, M.P.P., Janet Y. Rinehart, Ann Whelan, and Danna Korn. Special thanks to my original testers and tasters for lending their discerning palates to this project. They gave me valuable input about the dishes in this book in terms of taste, texture, and appearance.

The people who reviewed the original manuscript provided excellent feedback and offered many suggestions for improvement. They include Jane Dennison-Bauer, Maura Zazenski, Nancy Carol Sanker, O.T.R., Ellen Speare, C.N., Brett Fenster, M.D., and Kay DuBois. Since then, many others, too numerous to mention, have contributed invaluable suggestions. Thanks to each of you. I am grateful to John Duff, Laura Shepherd, Eileen Bertelli, Amy Tecklenburg, Rebecca Behan, and Kristen Jennings at Avery for their invaluable feedback on the book at various stages of the way, and to Jeanette Egan for creatively putting it all together.

My late friend, Jean Yancey, an accomplished businesswoman in her own right, was a continual source of ideas, encouragement, and support. Thank you, Jean! I miss you. And I am enormously grateful to Lisa Ekus, my wonderful, inspiring agent, for her guidance, support, and unflagging enthusiasm for my work.

Finally, a very special thank-you to Larry and Brett, my husband and son, who tasted dishes for the original edition, offered suggestions, and were very supportive, loving, and generous with their time. And our family now includes daughter-in-law, Helke, and grandson, Keene.

Contents

Preface

If there is such a thing as an accidental cookbook author, that would be me!

Writing cookbooks—especially wheat-free cookbooks—was not part of my life plan. But life is full of ironies, isn't it?

You see, I'm the daughter of a Nebraska farmer, a farmer who raised wheat. Wheat was a good thing at our house. It put food on the table and paid for my college tuition. After college, I married into a wheat-farming family. In fact, that's all they raise on their farm in western Nebraska. Furthermore, my father-in-law is an internationally known professor emeritus of agronomy at the University of Nebraska. What is his main area of expertise? You guessed it—wheat!

The irony is that wheat caused my lifetime struggle with nasal congestion and stuffiness, making me feel dull, groggy, and lethargic. For decades, I was plagued by chronic sinus infections requiring endless rounds of antibiotics. It always seemed like I was "coming down with a cold," and my sinus infections were often accompanied by laryngitis and bronchitis. And my eighty-hour workweek as a corporate marketing executive—interspersed with far too much transcontinental travel—didn't help.

It took several decades to discover that wheat is my nemesis and that I'm part of the 10 to 15 percent of Americans who can't eat it. In fact, when I was diagnosed, I kept hoping the doctor was wrong and that he would eventually call me to say it was all a big mistake! To make matters worse, I didn't know anyone else who couldn't eat wheat so I felt very isolated. And, of course, my new wheat-free way of life was puzzling to my wheat-farming family!

Before my diagnosis I never suspected wheat as the culprit behind my ill health. I didn't understand that it was the proteins in wheat—particularly gluten—that can be toxic to many of us. I didn't associate my fondness for baked goods—bagels, fresh-baked bread, pasta, cakes, and cookies—with the chronic congestion. And I had no idea that wheat lurked in the most unsuspecting places, such as licorice candy. Or that wheat is actually related to barley, rye, spelt, and kamut, all of which also must be avoided. After my diagnosis, I knew I had to take complete control of what I ate if I wanted to regain my health.

Life Takes a Turn

So, I began researching how I could prepare the same dishes I was accustomed to eating without wheat. I learned which alternative flours fit my diet and how these flours perform in various recipes. Eventually, I totally revamped my family's repertoire of dishes, and after a great deal of what my daughter-in-law calls "dishes, discourse, and discovery," I mastered the gluten-free lifestyle. I didn't know it yet, but I was starting down the path to being a cookbook author.

At the same time, my research revealed that millions of other people must also avoid wheat. I wasn't alone! Others were also forced to recognize and admit that we cannot continue to eat gluten and expect to feel good. I slowly came to realize that they also needed help in mastering the gluten-free lifestyle. I decided to turn my recipes into a cookbook so others could live successfully without gluten, too.

I wrote this book to help us all eat well without wheat or any of its noxious cousins—barley, rye, spelt, kamut, triticale—so each recipe is gluten-free, not just wheat-free. This book shows you how to adopt a gluten-free diet so you, too, can feel better—and still eat the dishes you want.

Cookbook Authors Are Made, Not Born

Before you read any further, it's important to set the record straight. It is true that I have a home economics degree, but I didn't study cooking. And it is true that I am now an accomplished cook, but I wasn't always so confident in the kitchen. In fact, I didn't even own a cookbook until I had been married three years. Until then, my method of cooking was "a little of this, a little of that," based on my mother's cooking style. Looking back, I had my share of disasters, too.

One particularly memorable near-catastrophe occurred one day when I was making a coffee-flavored whipped cream filling for a Mocha Brownie Torte. (I know it sounds exotic, but it was just coffee-flavored whipped cream sandwiched between two layers of brownies.) As I beat instant coffee powder into the heavy cream with a handheld electric mixer, I put my nose close to the bowl to see if the whipped cream smelled like coffee (which I love). My long hair caught in the beaters and before I knew it my hair was wrapped tightly around them, slamming the mixer against my head while the beaters rhythmically pounded at my scalp. Luckily, I quickly unplugged the mixer with my free hand, but the damage was done. Looking in the mirror as I carefully cut my hair out of the beaters, I felt lucky that this was my only injury!

Gluten-Free: New Diet for the Twenty-first Century

A lot has changed since I wrote the first edition of this book in 1995. Back then, the gluten-free diet was considered unusual. Celiac disease was virtually unknown to the general public. The medical community didn't pay much attention to celiac disease, labeling it a "rare" condition. Mainstream manufacturers, restaurants, and other businesses in the food industry barely acknowledged the gluten-free diet, leaving the field wide open for a handful of specialized entrepreneurs who tried to fill the void with cookbooks, mixes, and a few ready-made foods.

Today, the gluten-free diet is IN! Leading universities such as the University of Maryland, Columbia, Stanford, and the University of Chicago have established celiac research centers. Restaurants offer gluten-free dishes, new gluten-free foods appear on grocery shelves or are available from an extensive array of online vendors, and in August 2003, NBC's *Today* show featured a segment on celiac disease.

Specialized magazines such as *Gluten-Free Living* and *Living Without: A Lifestyle Guide for People with Food and Chemical Sensitivities* offer gluten-free advice. My cookbooks have been joined by others, so that we all have choices when we cook at home.

Finally, in 2003 leaders in the gluten-free community formed the American Celiac Task Force (www.celiaccenter.org/taskforce.asp) to present a unified voice to government, the food industry, and the public.

If there was ever a time to be gluten-free, it's now.

Carol Fenster, Ph.D.

Wheat-Free Recipes & Menus

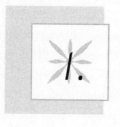

I. Introduction to Wheat-Free Cooking

Why Not Wheat?

Ordinarily, wheat is a very nutritious grain, and its marvelous baking properties make it our country's grain of choice. However, there are many reasons why wheat and its gluten-containing cousins may not be appropriate for everyone. Each of you reading this right now has a unique story, but basically most of you will fall into one of the following categories.

CELIAC DISEASE

Celiac disease is an inherited autoimmune disorder that affects the digestive process of the small intestine. When a person who has celiac disease consumes gluten—a protein found in wheat, rye, and barley—the individual's immune system responds by attacking the small intestine and inhibiting the absorption of important nutrients into the body.

Undiagnosed and untreated, celiac disease can lead to the development of other autoimmune disorders as well as osteoporosis, infertility, neurological conditions, and in rare cases, cancer (University of Chicago Celiac Disease Program, Facts and Figures, 2003). Another form of the disease is dermatitis herpetiformis (DH), with symptoms of skin rashes and blisterlike spots.

Celiac disease is far more common than originally thought. Once deemed "extremely rare," recent research by the Center for Celiac Research at the University of Maryland shows that approximately 1 in 133 Americans has celiac disease. This means that 2.2 million Americans are living with this disease, which takes an average of eleven years to get a correct diagnosis (Green, P. H., et al., "Characteristics of adult celiac disease in the U.S.A.: results of a national survey," *American Journal of Gastroenterology,* 2001).

Interestingly, this condition is much more common than many other diseases that get far more attention. For example, according to the University of Chicago Celiac Disease Program (quoting from the National Institutes of Health), celiac disease affects more people than those with Alzheimer's (2 million), Parkinson's disease (500,000), rheumatoid arthritis (2.1 million), or multiple sclerosis (333,000). Unlike these other diseases, however, there is no pill, no vaccine, and no surgical procedure. The only treatment is a gluten-free diet for life.

People with celiac disease must avoid *all* forms of gluten, which is present in wheat and wheat-related grains such as barley, rye, spelt, oats (possibly), and the less familiar grains of kamut and triticale.

Celiac disease is a lifelong condition that requires *strict* adherence to a gluten-free diet. Even people who don't exhibit the typical symptoms (diarrhea, bloating, gas, or fatigue), can still damage their intestines if they ingest gluten.

This condition must be managed with the help of a gastroenterologist, who performs a series of tests, including a small-bowel endoscopy while the patient is sedated, before a final diagnosis can be made. For more information on celiac disease, see Resources (page 251).

INTOLERANCES AND ALLERGIES

According to the Food Allergy & Anaphylaxis Network (FAAN), 2 to 2.5 percent of the general population suffers from food allergies, or about 6 to 7 million Americans. Wheat is one of the top eight food allergens affecting these allergic individuals.

True food allergies involve the immune system, and reactions are usually sudden and more pronounced. For example, I know of a young man who is so allergic to wheat that he had an anaphylactic reaction after entering a kitchen while somebody was baking. He apparently ingested some wheat flour particles that were floating through the air and was rushed to the emergency room for treatment after using his Epi-Pen to buy him more time. Few people have this type of severe allergy, but for those who do, it's *very* serious.

In contrast to the *few* people with wheat allergies, far more people, approximately 10 to 15 percent of Americans, have intolerances to wheat or gluten (*Clinical and Diagnostics Laboratory Immunology,* Vol. 7, 2000). In contrast to true food allergies, reactions involved in food intolerances *may* be delayed and are usually more subtle. My reaction to gluten is classified as an intolerance. In my case, my nasal stuffiness might be faintly apparent by the end of a wheat-laden meal yet be full-blown congestion by the next morning.

The reactions involved in food intolerances can take many different forms. Some people, like me, experience nasal congestion and stuffiness, a feeling of fatigue, and what we affectionately call "brain fog." Others have headaches (sometimes migraines), stomachaches, rashes, achy joints, and a host of other maladies that are as easily associated with other ailments as with a food intolerance. That's why it's often difficult to pinpoint food intolerances.

Food intolerances won't kill you, but they certainly compromise the quality of your life. Furthermore, the treatment for the symptoms can be as devastating as the symptoms themselves. In my case, endless rounds of antibiotics had a profound and lasting effect on my digestive system.

Diagnosis of a food allergy or intolerance should be made by a board-certified allergist or a health professional who specializes in this area. There are a variety of tests and procedures used to confirm a diagnosis. Testing for food allergies and intolerances remains a somewhat controversial area and not all experts agree on a single approach. For more information on food allergies and intolerances, see Resources (pages 251–56, including the Food Allergy & Anaphylaxis Network and York Nutritional Laboratories).

AUTISM—A SPECIAL CASE OF INTOLERANCE

Approximately 1 in 160 children are estimated to have autism, a perplexing neurobiological disorder that seems to be rising (*Wall Street Journal,* July 2003). Several experts advocate a gluten-free, casein-free diet (casein is a milk protein) as part of the overall treatment (but not as a substitute for other treatment). Apparently, some autistic children don't process these proteins properly, and removing them from the diet helps their behavior. I am not an expert in autism, but many families use my gluten-free recipes to prepare food for their autistic children. For more information on autism and the gluten-free, casein-free diet, consult your physician. Several associations included in Resources provide information about autism. You'll find more specific information on the diet at www.gfcfdiet.com.

OTHER MEDICAL CONDITIONS THAT
REQUIRE A GLUTEN-FREE DIET

In addition to celiac disease, food allergies or intolerances, and autism, certain people avoid gluten for other reasons. For example, part of the treatment for various auto-immune conditions such as multiple sclerosis, rheumatoid arthritis, and lupus may include a gluten-free diet. People with food-triggered asthma are sometimes placed on gluten-free diets.

You should rely on your physician to determine whether or not a gluten-free diet is appropriate for you. But, if it is, this book will help you. All of the recipes in this book avoid wheat and wheat-related grains such as barley, rye, spelt, or kamut by using gluten-free flours and by specifying gluten-free substitutes for other ingredients as well. They also avoid oats. See page 5 for a discussion of oats.

What It Means to Live on a Gluten-Free Diet

Living gluten-free means being aware of everything you put in your mouth. But, once you learn the ropes, it becomes a way of life. I've been *totally* gluten-free for nearly ten years now, and I know that I eat a much healthier diet: more fresh fruits and vegetables, less processed meat, and fewer refined foods.

Awareness of everything you eat means knowing exactly what's in your food, which requires that you read labels and understand the meaning of the words on the ingredients list. For more information on hidden gluten, see Hidden Sources of Gluten (page 243) in the Appendix.

Finding Gluten-Free Ingredients

It can be a bit daunting to keep up with which ingredients are safe and which aren't. Some associations provide lists of commercial products that are known to be safe. You can order the Commercial Product Listing from the Celiac Sprue Association (402-CSA-4CSA) or the Tri-Counties Shopping List from Tri-County Celiac Sprue Group, 47829 Vistas Circle, Canton, MI 48788. Or, go to www.clanthompson.com or www.celiac.com for gluten-free diet information.

In addition, *Gluten-Free Living* magazine reviews the safety of various ingredients (see Resources, page 251).

In addition to the ingredients above, a few foods continue to generate questions. Here is a brief discussion on the latest knowledge about these issues.

OATS—THE CURRENT STATUS

Oats have traditionally been excluded from the gluten-free diet even though experts agree that oats do not inherently contain gluten. The explanation is that oats *may* be contaminated with wheat because the two crops are grown in the same field during consecutive years (called rotation) and because their remarkably similar-looking kernels can be intermingled in manufacturing.

Several studies show that oats are safe to eat on a gluten-free diet, at least on a short-term basis, but experts are reluctant to encourage eating oats on a regular basis because there are no studies documenting the long-term effects of oat consumption. Nor are any manufacturers willing to guarantee their oats as gluten-free. To be on the safe side, I don't use oats in any recipe in this book, and I don't recommend them to anyone on a gluten-free diet. Check with your physician about eating oats.

DISTILLED SPIRITS, VINEGAR, AND VANILLA

Except for wine, gin, and tequila, alcoholic beverages have traditionally been omitted from the gluten-free diet. However, a careful review of the process by which distilled spirits are made shows that scotch, bourbon, and other distilled spirits are safe because the gluten peptides cannot survive the distillation process. Of course, any alcoholic beverage that is made from gluten-containing grains and is not distilled—such as beer—still contains gluten.

Vinegar is another ingredient that has traditionally been suspect. Even if the vinegar is made with gluten-containing grains (which it probably isn't), the gluten in the grains cannot survive the distillation process. The same is true of vanilla. This means you can use regular vanilla (instead of alcohol-free) and enjoy salad dressings made with vinegar—unless, of course, vanilla or vinegar bother you for other reasons, such as a sensitivity to fermented foods. If so, you should avoid them. You *must* avoid malt vinegar, though. It contains gluten because the malt is added back in *after* the distillation process using barley for the flavoring. (For a thorough discussion of distilled spirits, vanilla, and vinegar, see *Gluten-Free Living* magazine, Sept./Oct. and Nov./Dec. 1999, and Vol. 8, no. 3, 2003.)

Type of Dishes in this Book

Since this book is based on my own repertoire of recipes, it reflects my heritage and the culture in which I live. You'll see my midwestern roots reflected in dishes such as meat loaf or ham and scalloped potatoes. I've also traveled abroad and learned to appreciate many other cuisines, some of which are reflected in my recipes.

I've lived in Colorado for thirty years and have adopted (actually fallen in love with) southwestern cuisine, so you'll see many dishes with seasonings typical of Mexican food, such as chiles, cumin, lime juice, or oregano. This cuisine is very popular all across the country; famous chefs such as Rick Bayless, Bobby Flay, and others have built their careers on it. Southwestern cuisine also lends itself to gluten-free dishes because so many of them are based on corn rather than wheat and are very flavorful.

However, some people fear that boldly spiced southwestern food will have a negative impact on their digestive systems, especially those with celiac disease. If you've never eaten highly spiced food or if you know it disagrees with you, by all means avoid it. However, many people with celiac disease enjoy southwestern-style food with no ill effects. Nonetheless, if you choose to avoid this type of cuisine, relax; you'll find many other flavorful choices in this book.

To Your Health

Fortunately, the gluten-free community is broadening its focus from concern only with safety ("Does it contain gluten?") to include a growing interest in nutrition as well. For example, today's gluten-free consumers want to know the nutrient content of their food, so all the recipes in this book have been analyzed using MasterCook software and provide information for each recipe on calories, fat, protein, carbohydrate, fat, sodium, cholesterol, and fiber.

You'll find the nutrient content at the bottom of each recipe. These values are based on the U.S. Department of Agriculture (USDA) guidelines and are only approximate, since exact nutrient values may vary according to the size of a serving or to the particular brands of ingredients used.

Also, some of these values are rounded according to the Food and Drug Administration (FDA) guidelines. For example, if there are fewer than 5 grams of fat, the value is rounded to the nearest ½ gram. If more than 5 grams of fat, the value is rounded to the nearest whole number. Carbohydrates, proteins, sodium, and cholesterol are rounded to the nearest whole number. Calories are rounded to the nearest 5 calories. Fiber is rounded to the nearest ½ gram.

When there is more than one choice of ingredients, the analysis has been performed using the first choice. When a choice of flour blends is given, the nutrient content is based on Carol's Sorghum–Corn Flour Blend (page 11), my preferred blend for all gluten-free baking.

Some consumers also want healthy fats rather than hydrogenated versions. So, my recipes use healthy oils such as canola or olive oil and require only the minimum amount needed to produce a tasty dish. In each recipe that uses margarine or shortening, a non-hydrogenated, trans fat–free substitute is suggested.

Each recipe is gluten-free, but occasionally you will need to select a gluten-free version of a particular ingredient. For example, some brands of chicken broth contain wheat, but gluten-free versions exist. The term *gluten-free* in front of the ingredient means you must find a gluten-free brand of chicken broth.

Because lactose intolerance is one of the most common food sensitivities in America and because the ability of many people with celiac disease to digest lactose is impaired (especially during the early healing stages), I offer suggestions for dairy substitutes for milk, butter, and cheese in all recipes except those that must be dairy-based to work properly. When you need to choose a dairy-free version of an ingredient, it is preceded by the term *dairy-free.*

Stocking the Gluten-Free Pantry

Before you head into the kitchen, realize that some of the ingredients used in this book may be new to you. Most of you are probably familiar with wheat flour. But in this book you'll find other flours made from grains and vegetables that you probably didn't know could be made into flour, including sorghum, beans, rice, corn, tapioca, or potatoes, to mention just a few. And you'll learn about extremely nutritious flours you may never have heard of such as amaranth, quinoa, teff, or Indian rice grass (called Montina).

In addition to gluten-free flours, we use other ingredients that may be new to you, or used in ways you never thought of, such as dry milk powder, egg replacer, unflavored gelatin powder, and a few others. Each plays a vital, sometimes critical, role in the success of gluten-free cooking.

Stocking the gluten-free pantry is similar to stocking any pantry but with some different ingredients. In addition to the usual sugar, salt, pepper, and your favorite spices, below is a list of ingredients you'll want to have on hand so you're prepared for gluten-free cooking. These ingredients are not listed in order of importance but alphabetized instead. Beside each ingredient is a brief explanation of how you'll use it. Your pantry will expand as you discover other essential items.

Ingredients for the Gluten-Free Pantry	
INGREDIENT	**ROLE**
Baking powder, baking soda, cream of tartar	Leavens baked goods.
Butter, shortening, margarine, cooking oil	Adds fat to baked goods; use to grease baking pans.
Dry milk powder (This is not Carnation instant milk granules. I use Better Than Milk or Solait brand, which is a fine powder.)	Adds protein, which improves the texture of bread and provides food for yeast in baked goods.

Ingredients for the Gluten-Free Pantry

INGREDIENT	ROLE
Egg Replacer Powder (Ener-G Foods or Kingsmill)	Fine white powder that improves structure and texture of baked goods; adds leavening.
Flours: Sorghum, rice, garbanzo/fava bean, corn, white bean, potato starch, cornstarch, tapioca, arrowroot, almond, chestnut, and sweet rice	Use to create custom flour blends for baking; thickens sauces, gravies, and puddings.
Gelatin powder (unflavored) (Knox or Grayslake brands)	Adds moisture and protein to baked goods; binds ingredients.
Lecithin granules (Made of soy, it is available in the supplement section of health food stores.)	Yellowish-looking granules that improve texture and emulsify (combine) ingredients by binding oil and water.
Pasta in all shapes/sizes (My favorite is penne.)	Use in casseroles, pasta dishes, soups.
Vinegar	"Sours" milk into buttermilk. Serves as acidic food for yeast.
Xanthan gum, guar gum	Prevents crumbling in baked goods; thickens sauces and salad dressings. Either one or both are absolutely essential for successful gluten-free baking.
Yeast, dry active (Don't use rapid-rise yeast unless the recipe calls for it.)	Leavens baked goods and adds yeast flavor.

Gluten-Free Cooking Requires New, Innovative Techniques

In addition to new ingredients, you'll find new techniques that seem to defy conventional kitchen wisdom:

- using an electric mixer to beat the soft, sticky gluten-free dough rather than kneading it with your hands,
- putting bread dough in a *cold* rather than preheated *hot* oven, and
- mixing muffins with an electric mixer until they're well blended instead of using the usual "muffin method" of adding liquid ingredients into the "well" of dry ingredients and stirring just until blended.

EQUIPMENT AND ACCESSORIES

To cook using these sometimes "unconventional" cooking methods, you'll need the following utensils and other apparatus. Again, these items are alphabetized rather than listed in order of importance.

- Nonstick (gray color, not black) loaf pans, baking sheets, and pie pans: Gluten-free foods sometimes stick to the pan, so nonstick pans are a must, plus they brown food better than other pans.
- Plastic wrap, foil, waxed paper, paper towels: Cover food; aid in handling and shaping dough and batter.
- Parchment paper (silicone-lined paper): Line baking sheets for quick release of baked goods as well as easy cleanup.
- Stand mixer (I use a 4.5-quart KitchenAid): A heavy-duty mixer is useful for beating heavy, gluten-free dough and batter.

MIXING IT UP!

Gluten-free baking requires a blend of flours rather than just one flour (because no single flour will perform like wheat flour in baking). To simplify your baking, I provide three choices of gluten-free flour blends to use in the recipes in this book. Mix them up, store in a dark, dry place, and when you're ready to bake—you measure just once.

I personally prefer using the sorghum corn flour blend and I sometimes use the bean flour blend, but I know that there are many of you who still prefer to use rice flour–based blends, so I've also included a rice version. However, I strongly recommend that you try the sorghum corn flour blend. It's mildly flavored, produces baked goods with taste and texture superior to those made with rice, and provides a somewhat healthier dose of nutrients. Plus, rice flour blends can have a slightly gritty texture that the other blends don't have.

Store the flour blend in a large, heavy-duty plastic bag, a flour canister, or a large, screw-top glass jar with a wide mouth (my preference).

Carol's Sorghum–Corn Flour Blend

MAKES 4½ CUPS

1½ cups sorghum flour
1½ cups potato starch or cornstarch
1 cup tapioca flour
½ cup corn flour

To make the corn flour, grind white corn-meal (Quaker or Hodgson Hills), using a small coffee or spice grinder.

■ ■ ■

Carol's Bean Flour Blend

MAKES 4½ TO 5 CUPS

2½ cups garbanzo/fava bean flour
¾ cup potato starch or cornstarch
¾ cup tapioca flour
½ cup sorghum flour

■ ■ ■

Carol's Rice Flour Blend

MAKES 4½ TO 5 CUPS

2¾ cups brown rice flour
1¼ cups potato starch or cornstarch
¾ cup tapioca flour

■ ■ ■

FAVISM

If you're considering using the bean flour blend, you should know about favism. Favism is a rare genetic deficiency of the enzyme glucose-6-phophate dehydrogenase (G6PD). It is more prevalent among individuals of Mediterranean descent. Individuals who are G6PD-deficient can cause severe damage to red blood cells and subsequent anemia if they eat fava beans. One out of five people with this deficiency develops symptoms such as fatigue, shortness of breath, and an irregular heartbeat, usually after eating raw or partially cooked fava beans.

L-Dopa and Fava Beans

Fava beans (also called broad beans) contain L-dopa. People with Parkinson's disease may have symptoms aggravated by fava bean consumption, and people taking medications containing L-dopa should know that fava bean consumption can increase L-dopa levels excessively. Therefore, Parkinson's patients should speak with a doctor before adding fava beans to their diet. Despite these concerns, I have yet to meet anyone who can't use the extremely popular bean flour blends. Nonetheless, I want you to be forewarned.

WHERE YOU CAN FIND THESE INGREDIENTS

All of these ingredients are readily available at your local health food store. Sorghum flour is made by Authentic Foods, Bob's Red Mill, Ener-G Foods, and Twin Valley Mills. Or you can order by mail. [See the Appendix (page 257) for mail-order addresses.] The garbanzo/fava bean flour is available at health food stores from all the above companies, except Twin Valley Mills.

Secrets to Success with Gluten-Free Baking

Today, I still have some mini disasters, but I've learned a lot of secrets that I share with you in this book. If you follow these general guidelines, your baked goods—whether you're baking cakes, cookies, breads, or anything else—will turn out just fine. You'll find more baking tips specific to bread, an area about which I get lots of questions, in the next chapter.

A combination of gluten-free flours produces a better texture than single flours. For example, brown rice flour, when combined with potato starch and tapioca flour, is far less gritty than brown rice flour used alone. Always use a blend of flours in your baking.

Measure the flour by stirring it first to aerate it. Place the measuring cup on the counter. Spoon the flour into it, but don't pack it down. Using the straight edge of a knife, level the flour even with the top of the cup. This is the method used in developing all of the recipes in this book.

If you choose instead to dip the measuring cup into the flour and level it off by pressing it against the inside of the bag you will actually add 1 to 2 tablespoons more flour per cup than the recipe needs. We call this the "dip-and-sweep" method of measuring, and using it could negatively affect the results of your baking.

Smaller recipes (those containing 2 cups of flour or less) are easier to adapt to gluten-free flours. Recipes containing cake flour are especially easy to adapt because they don't depend upon gluten for their structure.

Gluten-free flours may require more leavening to compensate for their lack of elasticity. As a general rule, if you're converting your own recipes to gluten-free, use about 25 percent more baking soda or baking powder than in the wheat version. However, it usually isn't necessary to increase the yeast in yeast breads.

If your recipe calls for yeast, dissolve the yeast in the liquid portion of the recipe before adding it to the rest of the ingredients. This helps the bread rise better because the yeast will start rising sooner. In some recipes, especially flatbreads, which don't have to rise as much, you can just add the yeast along with the dry ingredients.

Parchment paper is an excellent way to prevent baked goods such as cookies from sticking to the baking sheet.

Remember that oven temperatures can vary tremendously from oven to oven. Buy a good oven thermometer and check the temperature of your oven.

STORAGE OF GLUTEN-FREE BAKED GOODS

Gluten-free baked goods are usually best warm from the oven. Because home-baked items don't have preservatives, their shelf life is short. It's best to refrigerate baked goods to prolong their freshness, but most of us can't eat the entire batch before its shelf life expires.

Therefore, many cooks cut baked items such as bread into individual slices, insert waxed paper between the slices, and freeze them, tightly wrapped. Frozen baked goods, especially breads and muffins, should be thawed at room temperature or gently heated at 30% in a microwave oven until defrosted. Using a microwave on full power (100%) to defrost baked goods makes them rubbery and tough.

2. The Gluten-Free Breadbasket: Yeast Breads, Quick Breads & Flatbreads

I n my opinion, nothing delights the senses better than a loaf of freshly baked bread. Before I went gluten-free, I baked my favorite cracked-wheat bread every weekend. Eager to taste it, I would slice off the crusty end piece as soon as it came out of the oven and slather it with butter. Along with a cup of freshly brewed coffee, I savored every single bite. I was in heaven!

Today, I still bake loaves of bread—and bagels, bread sticks, and focaccia—but they're gluten-free now. It took much mixing, baking, and tasting to master the intricacies of baking gluten-free breads, but I've taken the guesswork out for you by sharing my secrets in this chapter.

How Do Gluten-Free Breads Compare with Regular Bread

Breads made with gluten-free flours may look, taste, and smell slightly different from those made with wheat flour. Several reasons account for these differences, although, as our gluten-free ingredients and techniques improve over the years, these differences are less apparent.

First, breads made from gluten-free flours may look somewhat different. These flours do not have the same kinds of proteins needed to form the gluten framework that holds the gases that enable the bread to rise. As a result, these nonwheat breads may not be as large in volume or as light in texture as wheat breads. However, you will quickly come to appreciate their texture, and soon they'll seem totally familiar.

Second, gluten-free flours may taste slightly different because our taste buds have been conditioned to associate the "wheat" taste with bread. We've learned to expect the taste of wheat in bread. Gradually, your palate will come to expect and appreciate these newly acquired tastes.

Finally, the aroma we commonly associate with wheat bread is somewhat different. Rice flour has a unique aroma when it's baking, as does bean flour. Read "The Wonderful World of Gluten-free Flours" (page 233) to see how to use alternative flours, all of which are wonderful additions to our repertoire of flours. You'll find many of these flours in health food stores, If not, order them from the companies listed under Mail-Order Sources (page 257).

In this chapter, you'll find recipes for gluten-free breads that closely resemble "regular" breads. These recipes use ingredients that may be unfamiliar to help improve the volume, texture, flavor, and aroma of gluten-free breads. For example, xanthan gum provides structure to help trap the gases from yeast, baking powder, or baking soda and egg replacer (a commercial powder with leavening agents) improves the texture of breads.

Bread Machines Make Gluten-Free Bread Easy

New advances in technology, such as bread machines, can really streamline the bread-making process. With programmable machines, some experimentation may be required when using these recipes to achieve the right settings. My old, trusty Welbilt bread machine makes a great 1-pound loaf. I use the light setting. The machine warms the ingredients for 20 minutes, mixes for 10 minutes, rests for 5 minutes, kneads for 15 minutes, lets the dough rise for 25 minutes, punches down the dough, then lets it rise again for 54 minutes. It bakes for 40 minutes. The total time is 2 hours and 50 minutes. If you wish to program your machine for one rise, eliminate the second rise of 54 minutes. The bread recipes in this chapter are appropriate for bread machines making 1-pound and 1½-pound loaves.

Secrets to Successful Gluten-Free Bread Baking

In addition to the general guidelines for successful gluten-free baking in the first chapter, here are some more helpful hints.

- Dissolve the yeast in the combined liquid ingredients before adding it to the remaining ingredients in the recipe. This helps the bread rise.
- Add some form of protein—dry milk powder, eggs, soy lecithin granules, or unflavored gelatin powder—to improve the structure of yeast breads. Yeast needs protein to rise well.
- Let the dough rise just to the top of the loaf pan, no higher, before baking. It will continue to rise during baking.
- Bake the bread in smaller (5 x 3-inch rather than 9 x 5-inch), nonstick, gray (not black), loaf pans for better texture and more even baking. For nicely shaped sandwich slices and more stable loaves, bake 1-pound (8 x 4-inch loaves) rather than 1½-pound (9 x 5-inch loaves) recipes.
- Cover the bread with foil after the first 10 to 15 minutes of baking to avoid overbrowning.
- Bake breads at lower temperatures for longer periods of time, rather than higher temperatures for shorter baking periods. Most gluten-free breads are better when baked this way.
- Some bakers prefer to use filtered water rather than chlorinated water because chlorine can have an adverse effect on yeast.

Making Sandwiches from Gluten-Free Bread

We all enjoy a tasty sandwich now and then. There are several tricks to enhancing gluten-free bread to make it work even better for sandwiches. Here are a few tips:

- Lightly toast the bread to impart a deeper flavor and make it less likely to crumble. This technique works especially well for sandwiches that have "soggy" fillings, such as tuna salad or egg salad.
- Place hamburger buns, cut side down, on the grill for just a few minutes to lightly toast them and impart a slightly smoky flavor.
- Gently reheat bread slices, muffins, or flatbreads in the microwave oven on a low (perhaps 30%) power setting to restore moisture and pliability.
- Make grilled sandwiches such as a Reuben sandwich. These sandwiches are cooked on both sides (one side first, then the other) in a hot skillet. The grilling process seals and browns the bread and makes it firm and crisp. Grilling also imparts a deeper flavor.
- Purchase a sandwich grill or panini machine. This operates something like a waffle iron, which, when closed, cooks both sides of the sandwich simultaneously. The machine also presses the sandwich slightly, making it more compact and cohesive.

Bagels

Surprisingly easy to make, these are best eaten warm from the oven. A "schmear" of cream cheese enhances a breakfast bagel. Or, use your favorite deli fixin's to make a hearty sandwich.

MAKES 8 BAGELS

2½ cups flour blend (page 11)

½ cup potato starch

½ cup dry milk powder or nondairy milk powder

1 tablespoon active dry yeast

2 teaspoons xanthan gum

1 teaspoon guar gum

1 teaspoon salt

¾ cup warm water (110°F)

2 tablespoons canola oil

3 tablespoons honey

1 teaspoon cider vinegar

1 large egg, lightly beaten

1 teaspoon sugar

1 egg, beaten until foamy, for wash (optional)

1. Grease a large baking sheet or line with parchment paper. Combine all the ingredients, except the sugar and egg wash, in a large bowl. Beat with an electric mixer on low speed until well blended. Increase the speed to medium and beat for 2 minutes. The dough will be thick and stiff, but also very sticky.

2. Place the dough on a flat, white rice-floured surface. Divide it into 8 equal portions. Dust each portion with rice flour to make it easier to handle; and shape into balls. Flatten the balls to 3-inch circles and punch a hole in the center of each, continuing to dust with rice flour, if necessary, to prevent sticking. Form into bagel shapes, turning the rough edges of dough to the undersides. Be sure to make the hole at least 1½ inches in diameter because the hole will grow smaller as the dough rises.

3. Place the bagels on the prepared baking sheet. Place the bagels in a cold oven; turn the oven temperature control to 325°F. Bake for 15 minutes. Remove the bagels from the oven, but leave the oven on. The bagels may look a little rough at this stage, but they will become smoother during the boiling and final baking.

4. Meanwhile, bring 3 inches of water and the sugar to a boil in a deep skillet or Dutch oven. Boil the bagels for 30 seconds on each side. Grease the baking sheet again if you're not using parchment paper. Return the bagels to the baking sheet. For a nice sheen, brush the bagels with the egg wash.

5. Return the bagels to the oven and increase the oven temperature to 400°F. Bake for 20 to 25 minutes, or until the bagels are nicely browned. If the bagels brown too quickly, cover them with aluminum foil. Remove the bagels from the baking sheet and cool on a wire rack.

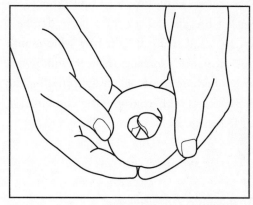

Forming a Bagel

Per bagel
CALORIES: 315 FAT: 5g PROTEIN: 5g CARBOHYDRATES: 65g SODIUM: 298mg CHOLESTEROL: 23mg FIBER: 1g

VARIATION

Cinnamon Bagels
Add 2 teaspoons cinnamon and ½ cup raisins in step 1.

Per bagel
CALORIES: 345 FAT: 5g PROTEIN: 5g CARBOHYDRATES: 73g SODIUM: 298mg CHOLESTEROL: 23mg FIBER: 1g

■ ■ ■

Bread Sticks

Serve these tasty bread sticks piled high in a wicker breadbasket, or for a more dramatic effect, stand them upright in a wide-mouth container. You can experiment by adding different herbs to the dough or by sprinkling the bread sticks with your favorite combination of Italian spices.

MAKES 10 BREAD STICKS

1 tablespoon active dry yeast

½ cup white or brown rice flour

½ cup tapioca flour

1 tablespoon dry milk powder or nondairy milk powder

2 teaspoons xanthan gum

½ cup grated Parmesan cheese (cow or soy)

½ teaspoon salt

1 teaspoon onion powder

1 teaspoon unflavored gelatin powder

⅔ cup warm water (110°F)

½ teaspoon sugar

1 tablespoon olive oil

1 teaspoon cider vinegar

Nonstick cooking spray (optional)

1 egg white, beaten to foamy (optional)

1 teaspoon Italian seasoning

1. Preheat the oven to 400°F for 5 minutes, then turn the heat off. Grease a large baking sheet or line with parchment paper.

2. While oven is preheating, in a medium bowl, blend the yeast, flours, milk powder, xanthan gum, Parmesan, salt, onion powder, and gelatin with an electric mixer on low speed. Add the water, sugar, oil, and vinegar. Increase the speed to high and beat for 2 minutes. The dough will be soft and sticky. (For easier preparation, add all the ingredients, except the egg white and Italian seasoning, to a food processor and blend until the mixture forms a soft ball.)

3. Cut a diagonal ½-inch opening on one corner (this makes a 1-inch circle) of a large, heavy-duty, resealable plastic freezer bag and place the dough in the bag. Squeeze the dough out of the plastic bag onto the prepared baking sheet in 10 strips, each 1 inch wide and 6 inches long. For the best results, hold the bag of dough upright as you squeeze, rather than at an angle, and position the seam of the bag on top, instead of at the side. For a glossy crust, spray the bread sticks with cooking spray or brush with the egg white, if desired, then sprinkle with the herb seasoning.

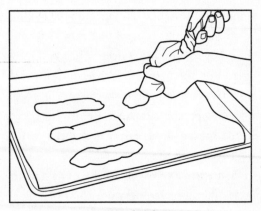

Breadsticks

4. Place the bread sticks in the oven with the heat off; let rise for 20 to 30 minutes until doubled in size.

5. Turn the oven temperature to 400°F and bake the bread sticks for 15 to 20 minutes, until golden brown, switching the position of the baking sheet halfway through baking to assure even browning. Cool on a wire rack. Store in an airtight container.

Per bread stick

CALORIES: 85 FAT: 3g PROTEIN: 3g CARBOHYDRATES: 13g SODIUM: 192mg CHOLESTEROL: 3mg FIBER: 1g

■ ■ ■

Crostini

This Italian favorite (pronounced crow-STEE-nee) is as versatile as you want to make it. When I was on a gluten-free culinary tour of Tuscany a few years ago, we ate it topped with fresh tomatoes or liver pâté. Feel free to experiment with your own toppings. With crostini, anything goes.

MAKES 4 (2-SLICE) SERVINGS

1 loaf French Bread (page 25)
2 tablespoons extra-virgin olive oil
1 garlic clove, minced
½ teaspoon salt
¼ cup grated Parmesan cheese (cow or soy)
2 tablespoons finely chopped fresh parsley
Suggested topping, optional (below)

1. Preheat the oven to 350°F. Grease a baking sheet or line with parchment paper. Cut the bread diagonally into about 24 (½-inch-thick) slices. The number of slices will vary with the size of the baguette, but it is important to keep the slices at a uniform thickness so they toast evenly in the oven.

2. Mix the oil, garlic, and salt in a small bowl. Use a pastry brush to coat one side of each slice with the oil mixture and place on coated side up on the prepared baking sheet.

3. Bake for 5 minutes; turn each slice over and bake for 2 minutes to brown lightly on the undersides. The goal is very lightly toasted bread, so adjust the baking time and turn slices accordingly. Watch carefully so the bread doesn't burn. Sprinkle with the Parmesan and parsley and bake for about 1 minute longer, or until the cheese melts.

4. Arrange the hot bread on a serving plate. Top with one of the suggested toppings, if desired, and serve.

Per serving (without topping)

CALORIES: 100 FAT: 5g PROTEIN: 3g CARBOHYDRATES: 13g SODIUM: 500mg CHOLESTEROL: 5mg FIBER: 0.5g

TOPPINGS

Black-Olive Topping

In food processor, combine ¾ cup pitted black olives, 1 garlic clove, ⅛ teaspoon dried thyme, 1 teaspoon dried basil, and 1 teaspoon olive oil. Purée until smooth.

Additional Suggestions

Feta cheese, pesto, blue cheese, jam, or roasted onions

■ ■ ■

English Muffins

English Muffins are great toasted for breakfast or as the base for Eggs Benedict (page 204). They can also be used to make delicious, portable sandwiches that stand up well in lunch boxes.

MAKES 12 MUFFINS

2 tablespoons active dry yeast

1 tablespoon sugar

1 ¼ cups warm water (110°F)

2 ⅓ cups flour blend (page 11)

2 cups tapioca flour

⅔ cup dry milk powder or nondairy milk powder

1 tablespoon xanthan gum

1 tablespoon unflavored gelatin powder

1 teaspoon salt

¼ teaspoon potato flour (not potato starch)

¼ cup margarine (see note below)

4 large egg whites, at room temperature

1. Grease a baking sheet and dust with cornmeal. Dissolve the yeast and sugar in the water in a small bowl. Let stand for 5 minutes, or until foamy.

2. In a large mixer bowl, combine the flour blend, tapioca flour, dry milk, xanthan gum, gelatin, salt, and potato flour. Beat with an electric mixer on low speed until blended, then add the margarine and egg whites. Beat until well blended. Add the yeast mixture and beat on high speed for 2 minutes.

3. To make foil muffin rings, cut a 12-inch length of foil and fold in half, lengthwise, again and again, until the strip is 1 inch wide and 12 inches long. Secure the ends together with masking tape. (See drawings on page 23.) Repeat to make 12 rings. Spray the insides of the rings with cooking spray. Arrange the muffin rings on the prepared baking sheet.

4. Divide the dough into 12 equal pieces and press 1 piece into each ring. Cover and let rise in a warm place for about 50 minutes, or until the dough is level with the tops of the rings.

5. Preheat the oven to 350°F. Bake the muffins for 15 minutes, or until lightly browned. With a spatula, turn the muffins (rings and all) over and bake 10 minutes longer, or until lightly browned.

6. Remove the muffins from the baking sheet and cool on a wire rack. When the rings are cool enough to handle, remove the muffins from the rings.

Per muffin

CALORIES PER MUFFIN: 300 FAT: 5g PROTEIN: 6g CARBO-HYDRATES: 63g SODIUM: 237mg CHOLESTEROL: 1mg FIBER: 1g

Note: Nonhydrogenated trans fat-free margarines by Earth Balance or Spectrum are available at health food stores.

■ ■ ■

Aluminum Foil Rings for English Muffins: The Three Steps

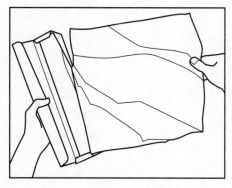

Step One

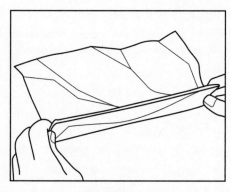

Step Two

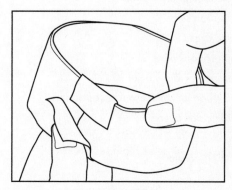

Step Three

Focaccia

Focaccia is a cross between pizza and rustic flat bread. It's easy to make, and the dough is especially forgiving. At serving time, dip it into flavored olive oil or spaghetti sauce, just like the Italian restaurants.

MAKES 10 SERVINGS

1 ½ teaspoons active dry yeast

1 teaspoon sugar

¾ cup warm water (110°F)

1 ½ cups flour blend (page 11)

½ cup tapioca flour

1 ½ teaspoons xanthan gum

1 teaspoon unflavored gelatin powder

1 teaspoon dried rosemary

½ teaspoon onion powder

1 teaspoon salt

2 large eggs

3 tablespoons olive oil

½ teaspoon cider vinegar

1 teaspoon Italian seasoning (optional)

1 tablespoon olive oil

TOPPING (below)

1. Grease an 11 x 7-inch nonstick pan. Dissolve the yeast and sugar in the water in a small bowl. Let stand for 5 minutes, or until foamy.

2. Combine the flour blend, tapioca flour, xanthan gum, gelatin, rosemary, onion powder, and ¾ teaspoon of the salt in a mixing bowl. Whisk the eggs, 2 tablespoons of the oil, and vinegar into the yeast mixture and stir into the dry ingredients. Beat the dough with an electric mixer on low speed for 2 minutes, using a spatula to keep stirring down the dough if it clings to the beaters. The dough will be soft and sticky

3. Transfer the dough to the prepared pan. Sprinkle with Italian seasoning, if using, the remaining ¼ teaspoon salt, and the remaining 1 tablespoon oil. Cover with aluminum foil and let rise in a warm place until not quite level with the top of the pan, 30 minutes. (If desired, omit the Italian seasoning and top with one of the toppings below.)

4. Preheat oven to 400°F. Bake for 15 to 20 minutes, until nicely browned.

Per serving

CALORIES: 150 FAT: 5g PROTEIN: 2g CARBOHYDRATES: 26g
SODIUM: 226mg CHOLESTEROL: 36mg FIBER: 0.5g

VARIATIONS

Herb Topping

Combine ½ teaspoon dried rosemary, ½ teaspoon dried sage, ½ teaspoon dried thyme, ¼ teaspoon black pepper, and 2 tablespoons Parmesan cheese (cow or soy).

Sun-Dried Tomato and Olive Topping

Combine ¼ cup chopped oil-packed sun-dried tomatoes, ¼ cup chopped pitted black olives, and ¼ cup chopped onion sautéed until translucent in 1 teaspoon olive oil.

Pesto Topping

Purée the following: In a food processor, combine 1 cup fresh basil leaves, 1 garlic clove, and ½ cup pine nuts and purée just until smooth, leaving a bit of texture. With motor running, slowly drizzle in ¼ cup olive oil through feed tube. Add ¼ cup grated Parmesan cheese (cow or soy) and a dash of freshly ground black pepper.

◼ ◼ ◼

French Bread

I know it sounds impossible, but you can have fresh bread hot from the oven in just an hour! This recipe is fast and has a crispy crust because it goes directly into a cold oven without any rising.

MAKES 2 LOAVES; 20 SLICES

2 tablespoons active dry yeast

1 tablespoon sugar

1¼ cups warm water (110°F)

2 cups Sorghum-Corn Flour Blend (page 11)

1 cup potato starch

¼ cup dry milk powder or nondairy
   milk powder

1 teaspoon guar gum

1 teaspoon xanthan gum

1½ teaspoons salt

1 tablespoon butter or margarine
   (see note, page 23), at room temperature

3 large egg whites, lightly beaten

1 teaspoon cider vinegar

1 egg white, beaten until foamy, for wash
   (optional)

1. Dissolve the yeast and sugar in the water in a small bowl. Let stand for 5 minutes, or until foamy.

2. Grease 2 French bread pans or line with parchment paper. (I like to use the perforated French bread pans, lined with parchment paper to prevent the dough from leaking through the perforations.)

3. In the bowl of a heavy-duty stand mixer, combine the flour blend, potato starch, milk powder, guar gum, xanthan gum, and salt. With the mixer on low speed, beat until blended. Add yeast mixture. On low speed, beat in the butter, egg whites, and vinegar, then beat on high speed for 2 minutes. The dough will be somewhat soft.

4. Spoon the dough into the prepared pans, shaping the dough into baguettes. Brush with the egg white wash for a glossier crust. Place immediately on the middle rack of a cold oven. Set the temperature to 425°F and bake for 30 to 35 minutes, until the bread is nicely browned. Cover with foil if the bread browns too quickly.

5. Remove the bread from the pans and cool completely on a wire rack. Slice with electric knife or serrated knife.

Per slice
CALORIES: 130 FAT: 1g PROTEIN: 2g CARBOHYDRATES: 30g SODIUM: 330mg CHOLESTEROL: 2mg FIBER: 1g

Note: You can place the dough in a French bread pan, let it rise to the top of the pan, and bake it in a preheated 425°F oven for 25 to 30 minutes, until nicely browned.

■ ■ ■

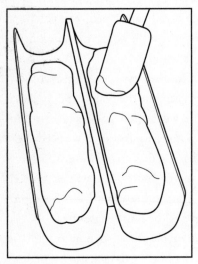

French Bread

Hamburger Buns

If you've eaten hamburger patties without a bun for so long that you've forgotten what a real hamburger tastes like, this recipe will definitely refresh your memory. They're especially good lightly toasted.

MAKES 8 BUNS

1 ½ teaspoons dry yeast
1 teaspoon sugar
1 ½ cups flour blend (page 11)
1 tablespoon instant chopped onion
1 ½ teaspoons xanthan gum
1 teaspoon unflavored gelatin powder
¾ teaspoon salt
¼ teaspoon soy lecithin granules
¾ cup warm water (110°F)
2 tablespoons canola oil
2 large eggs
½ teaspoon cider vinegar

1. Combine the yeast, sugar, flour blend, onion, xanthan gum, gelatin, salt, and lecithin in a bowl. Add the water, oil, eggs, and vinegar to the dry ingredients. Beat with an electric mixer at high speed, using regular beaters, not dough hook, for 2 minutes. The dough will be soft and sticky.

2. Spray a baking sheet and 8 foil rings (see page 22) with cooking spray and arrange the rings on the baking sheet. Divide the

dough into 8 equal pieces and press 1 piece into each ring. Cover with foil and let rise in a warm place for 30 minutes, or until level with the tops of the rings.

3. Preheat the oven to 400°F. Bake the buns for 15 to 20 minutes, until the tops are golden brown. Cool on a wire rack for 5 minutes, then remove the buns from the rings. To serve, cut horizontally in half and lightly toast cut sides of buns before serving for a crunchier texture.

Per bun

CALORIES: 205 FAT: 5g PROTEIN: 3g CARBOHYDRATES: 39g SODIUM: 216mg CHOLESTEROL: 45mg FIBER: 1g

VARIATION

For an herb-flavored bun, add 1 teaspoon crushed dried rosemary leaves and ½ teaspoon Italian seasoning in step 1.

▪ ▪ ▪

✳ Dilly Bread

This is my grandmother's recipe, which was passed down from my mother to me. I've modified it for gluten-free flours. Cottage cheese improves the structure of gluten-free breads and is important in this recipe, so it's not dairy-free.

MAKES EITHER A 1-POUND (12 SERVINGS) OR A 1½-POUND (18 SERVINGS) LOAF

	1-POUND LOAF (8 x 4-INCH PAN)	1½-POUND LOAF (9 x 5-INCH PAN)
Active dry yeast	2¼ teaspoons	2¼ teaspoons
Sugar	4 teaspoons	6 teaspoons
Water	¼ cup	10 tablespoons
Low-fat cottage cheese	1 cup	1½ cups
Large eggs, at room temperature	2	3
Canola oil	1 tablespoon	1½ tablespoons
Cider vinegar	1 teaspoon	1½ teaspoons
Flour blend (page 11)	2 cups	3 cups
Potato flour (*not* potato starch)	¼ teaspoon	½ teaspoon
Instant chopped onion	1 tablespoon	1½ tablespoons

Dried dill weed	1 tablespoon	1½ tablespoons
Dill seed	1 tablespoon	1½ tablespoons
Baking soda	¼ teaspoon	¼ heaping teaspoon
Salt	½ teaspoon	¾ teaspoon
Xanthan gum	2 teaspoons	1 tablespoon
Unflavored gelatin powder	1 teaspoon	1½ teaspoons

To make by hand:

1. Grease a loaf pan. Dissolve the yeast and 1 teaspoon of the sugar in warm water (110°F) in a small bowl. Set aside for 5 minutes, or until foamy. Warm the cottage cheese to room temperature.

2. In a large mixer bowl, combine the yeast mixture with the remaining ingredients, including the remaining sugar. With an electric mixer on low speed, using regular beaters not dough hook, slowly beat the ingredients until just blended. Increase the speed to high and beat for 2 minutes.

3. Transfer the dough to the prepared pan. Let rise in a warm place (75°F to 80°F) until the dough is level with the top of the pan.

4. Preheat the oven to 375°F. Bake for 45 to 50 minutes, until the loaf makes a clicking sound when tapped with your fingernail. Baking times can vary significantly; some loaves take less time; others more. Cover with foil if the bread browns too quickly. Cool in the pan on a wire rack for 5 minutes. Remove from the pan and finish cooling on wire rack.

To make in a bread machine:

1. Follow the bread machine instructions. [I usually combine the dry ingredients, then pour them into the bread machine. Then I combine the liquid ingredients (using water at room temperature) and pour them over the dry ingredients in the bread machine.]

2. Set controls and bake.

Per serving

CALORIES: 180 FAT: 2.5g PROTEIN: 6g CARBOHYDRATES: 35g SODIUM: 121mg CHOLESTEROL: 30mg FIBER: 1g

■ ■ ■

Fennel Bread

Fennel bread is dark, dense, and delicious. It tastes great in sandwiches but also lends a slightly exotic flavor when served with dinner.

MAKES EITHER A 1-POUND (12 SERVINGS) OR A 1½-POUND (18 SERVINGS) LOAF

	1-POUND LOAF (8 x 4-INCH PAN)	1½-POUND (9 x 5-INCH PAN)
Active dry yeast	2¼ teaspoons	2¼ teaspoons
Light brown sugar	3 tablespoons	¼ cup
Water	1 cup	1½ cups
Flour blend (page 11)	2⅛ cups	3¼ cups
Salt	1 teaspoon	1½ teaspoons
Xanthan gum	2 teaspoons	1 tablespoon
Unflavored gelatin powder	1 teaspoon	1½ teaspoons
Fennel seeds	1 tablespoon	1½ tablespoons
Flaxseeds (optional)	1 tablespoon	1½ tablespoons
Dry milk powder or nondairy milk powder	⅓ cup	½ cup
Potato flour (*not* potato starch)	¼ teaspoon	¼ heaping teaspoon
Soy lecithin	¼ teaspoon	¼ heaping teaspoon
Large eggs, lightly beaten	2	3
Canola oil	3 tablespoons	¼ cup
Cider vinegar	1 teaspoon	1½ teaspoons
Molasses	1 tablespoon	1½ tablespoons

To make by hand:

1. Grease a loaf pan. Dissolve the yeast and 2 teaspoons of the sugar in warm water (110°F) in a small bowl. Set aside for 5 minutes, or until foamy.

2. In a large mixer bowl, combine the yeast mixture with the remaining ingredients (including the remaining sugar). With an electric mixer on low speed, using regular beaters, not dough hooks, beat the ingredients just until blended. Increase the speed to high and beat for 2 minutes.

3. Transfer the dough to the prepared pan. Let rise in a warm place (75°F to 80°F) until the dough is level with the top of the pan.

4. Preheat the oven to 375°F. Bake for 45 to 50 minutes, until the loaf makes a clicking sound when tapped with your fingernail. Baking times can vary significantly; some loaves take less time, others more. Cover with foil if the bread browns too quickly. Cool in the pan on a wire rack for 5 minutes. Remove from the pan and finish cooling on wire rack.

To make in a bread machine:

1. Follow the bread machine instructions. [I usually combine the dry ingredients, then pour them into the bread machine. Then I combine the liquid ingredients (using water at room temperature) and pour them over the dry ingredients in the bread machine.]

2. Set controls and bake.

Per serving

CALORIES: 210 FAT: 4.5g PROTEIN: 4g CARBOHYDRATES: 41g SODIUM: 200mg CHOLESTEROL: 30mg FIBER: .5g

■ ■ ■

Pumpernickel Bread

This bread is thick, dense, and hearty. It's great for any sandwich, but especially good for a Reuben.

MAKES EITHER A 1-POUND (12 SERVINGS) OR A 1½-POUND (18 SERVINGS) LOAF

	1-POUND LOAF (8 x 4-INCH PAN)	1½-POUND LOAF (9 x 5-INCH PAN)
Active dry yeast	2¼ teaspoons	2¼ teaspoons
Light brown sugar	2 tablespoons	3 tablespoons
Water	1 cup	1½ cups
Flour blend (page 11)	2 cups	3 cups
Dry milk powder or nondairy milk powder	⅓ cup	½ cup
Unsweetened cocoa powder	1 tablespoon	1½ tablespoons
Caraway seeds	1 tablespoon	1½ tablespoons
Flaxseeds (optional)	1 teaspoon	2 teaspoons

Xanthan gum	2 teaspoons	3 teaspoons
Instant coffee powder	1 teaspoon	1 ½ teaspoons
Unflavored gelatin powder	1 teaspoon	1 ½ teaspoons
Salt	1 teaspoon	1 ½ teaspoons
Onion powder	½ teaspoon	¾ teaspoon
Potato flour (not potato starch)	¼ teaspoon	¼ heaping teaspoon
Large whole eggs, at room temperature	2	3
Canola oil	2 tablespoons	3 tablespoons
Molasses	2 tablespoons	3 tablespoons
Cider vinegar	1 teaspoon	1 ½ teaspoons
Grated orange zest (optional)	½ teaspoon	¾ teaspoon

To make by hand:

1. Grease a loaf pan. Dissolve the yeast and 2 teaspoons of the sugar in warm water (110°F) in a small bowl. Let stand for 5 minutes, or until foamy.

2. In a large mixer bowl, combine yeast mixture with remaining ingredients (including the remaining sugar). With the mixer on low speed, using regular beaters, not dough hooks, slowly blend the ingredients together. Increase the speed to high and beat for 2 minutes.

3. Transfer the dough to the prepared pan. Let rise in a warm place (75°F to 80°F) until the dough is level with the top of the pan.

4. Preheat the oven to 375°F. Bake for 45 to 50 minutes, until the loaf makes a clicking sound when tapped with your fingernail. Baking times can vary significantly; some loaves take less time, others more. Cover with foil if bread browns too quickly. Cool in the pan on a wire rack for 5 minutes. Remove from the pan and finish cooling on wire rack.

To make in a bread machine:

1. Follow the bread machine instructions. [I usually combine the dry ingredients, then pour them into the bread machine. Then I combine the liquid ingredients, (using water at room temperature) and pour over the dry ingredients in the bread machine.]

2. Set controls and bake.

Per serving
CALORIES: 195 FAT: 4g PROTEIN: 4g CARBOHYDRATES: 39g SODIUM: 200mg CHOLESTEROL: 30mg FIBER: 1g

■ ■ ■

Raisin Bread

This makes a wonderful breakfast bread. Eat it plain or toasted, or with butter, jam, or cream cheese.

MAKES EITHER A 1-POUND (14 SERVINGS) OR A 1½-POUND (18 SERVINGS) LOAF

	1-POUND LOAF (8 x 4-INCH PAN)	1½-POUND LOAF (9 x 5-INCH PAN)
Active dry yeast	2¼ teaspoons	2¼ teaspoons
Granulated sugar	1 teaspoon	1½ teaspoons
Water	1 cup	1½ cups
Flour blend (page 11)	2 cups	3 cups
Dry milk powder or nondairy milk powder	⅓ cup	½ cup
Light brown sugar	2 tablespoons	3 tablespoons
Xanthan gum	1½ teaspoons	2½ teaspoons
Unflavored gelatin powder	1 teaspoon	1½ teaspoons
Salt	1 teaspoon	1½ teaspoons
Ground cinnamon	1 teaspoon	1½ teaspoons
Soy lecithin granules	¼ teaspoon	¼ heaping teaspoon
Large whole eggs, lightly beaten	2	3
Canola oil	3 tablespoons	¼ cup
Cider vinegar	1 teaspoon	1½ teaspoons
Applesauce or prune baby food	¼ cup	¼ cup plus 2 tablespoons
Raisins	½ cup	¾ cup

To make by hand:

1. Grease a loaf pan. Dissolve the yeast and granulated sugar in warm water (110°F) in a small bowl. Let stand for 5 minutes, or until foamy.

2. In a large mixer bowl, combine the yeast mixture with the remaining ingredients. With an electric mixer on low speed, using regular beaters, not dough hooks, slowly blend ingredients together. Increase speed to high and beat for 2 minutes.

3. Transfer the dough to the prepared pan. Let rise in a warm place (75°F to 80°F) until the dough is level with the top of the pan.

4. Preheat the oven to 375°F. Bake for 45 to 50 minutes, until the loaf makes a clicking sound when tapped with your fingernail. Baking times can vary significantly; some loaves take less time, others more. Cover with foil if bread browns too quickly. Cool in the pan on a wire rack for 5 minutes. Remove from pan and finish cooling on wire rack.

To make in a bread machine:

1. Follow the machine instructions. [I usually combine the dry ingredients, then pour them into the bread machine. Then I combine the liquid ingredients (using water at room temperature) and pour over the dry ingredients in the bread machine.]

2. Set controls and bake.

Per serving

CALORIES: 215 FAT: 5g PROTEIN: 4g CARBOHYDRATES: 42g SODIUM: 200mg CHOLESTEROL: 30mg FIBER: 1g

■ ■ ■

Russian Black Bread

A dark, hearty bread that makes a great sandwich with tuna salad or smoked meats—or a Reuben.

MAKES EITHER A 1-POUND (12 SERVINGS) OR A 1½-POUND (18 SERVINGS) LOAF

	1-POUND LOAF (8 x 4-INCH PAN)	1½-POUND LOAF (9 x 5-INCH PAN)
Active dry yeast	2¼ teaspoons	2¼ teaspoons
Sugar	1 teaspoon	1½ teaspoons
Water	1 cup	1½ cups
Flour blend (page 11)	2 cups	3 cups
Fennel seeds	2 teaspoons	1 tablespoon
Flaxseeds	2 teaspoons	1 tablespoon
Instant coffee powder	2 teaspoons	1 tablespoon
Onion powder	½ teaspoon	¾ teaspoon

Xanthan gum	2 teaspoons	1 tablespoon
Salt	1 teaspoon	1 ½ teaspoons
Unflavored gelatin powder	1 teaspoon	1 ½ teaspoons
Potato flour (*not* potato starch)	¼ teaspoon	¼ heaping teaspoon
Dry milk powder or nondairy milk powder	⅓ cup	½ cup
Unsweetened cocoa powder	2 tablespoons	3 tablespoons
Large whole eggs, at room temperature	2	3
Canola oil	2 tablespoons	3 tablespoons
Cider vinegar	1 teaspoon	1 ½ teaspoons
Molasses	¼ cup	¼ cup plus 2 tablespoons

To make by hand:

1. Grease a loaf pan. Dissolve the yeast and sugar in warm water (110°F) in a small bowl. Let stand for 5 minutes, or until foamy.

2. In a large mixer bowl, combine the yeast mixture with the remaining ingredients. With an electric mixer on low speed, using regular beaters, not dough hooks, slowly beat the ingredients just until blended. Increase speed to high and beat for 2 minutes.

3. Transfer the dough to the prepared pan. Let rise in a warm place (75°F to 80°F) until the dough is level with the top of the pan.

4. Preheat the oven to 375°F. Bake for 45 to 50 minutes, until the loaf makes a clicking sound when tapped with your fingernail. Baking times can vary significantly. Cover with foil if bread browns too quickly. Cool in the pan on a wire rack for 5 minutes. Remove from the pan and finish cooling on wire rack.

To make in a bread machine:

1. Follow the bread machine instructions. [I usually combine the dry ingredients, then pour them into the bread machine. Then I combine liquid ingredients (using water at room temperature) and pour them over the dry ingredients in the bread machine.]

2. Set controls and bake.

Per serving
CALORIES: 200 FAT: 4g PROTEIN: 4g CARBOHYDRATES: 40g SODIUM: 202mg CHOLESTEROL: 30mg FIBER: 1g

■ ■ ■

Sandwich Bread

This is the trusty standby for sandwiches, toast, or bread crumbs. Stale leftovers make great croutons or bread pudding.

MAKES EITHER A 1-POUND (12 SERVINGS) OR A 1½-POUND (18 SERVINGS) LOAF

	1-POUND LOAF (8 x 4-INCH PAN)	1½-POUND LOAF (9 x 5-INCH PAN)
Active dry yeast	2¼ teaspoons	2¼ teaspoons
Sugar	2 tablespoons	2½ tablespoons
Water	1 cup	1½ cups
Flour blend (page 11)	2¼ cups	3⅓ cups
Dry milk powder or nondairy milk powder	⅓ cup	½ cup
Xanthan gum	2 teaspoons	1 tablespoon
Salt	1 teaspoon	1½ teaspoons
Soy lecithin granules	¼ teaspoon	¼ heaping teaspoon
Egg replacer powder	1 teaspoon	1½ teaspoons
Large whole eggs, lightly beaten	2	3
Melted butter or canola oil	3 tablespoons	¼ cup
Cider vinegar	1 teaspoon	1½ teaspoons

To make by hand:

1. Grease a loaf pan. Dissolve the yeast and 2 teaspoons of the sugar in warm water (110°F) in a small bowl. Let stand for 5 minutes, or until foamy.

2. In a large mixer bowl, combine the yeast mixture with the remaining ingredients (including remaining sugar). With an electric mixer on low speed, using regular beaters, not dough hooks, slowly beat ingredients until just blended. Increase speed to high and beat for 2 minutes.

3. Transfer the dough to the prepared pan. Let rise in a warm place (75°F to 80°F) until the dough is level with the top of the pan.

4. Preheat the oven to 375°F. Bake for 45 to 50 minutes, until the loaf makes a clicking sound when tapped with your fingernail. Baking times can vary significantly; some loaves take less time, others more. Cover with foil if bread browns too quickly. Cool in the pan on a wire rack for 5 minutes. Remove from the pan and finish cooling on wire rack.

To make in a bread machine:

1. Follow the bread machine instructions. [I usually combine the dry ingredients, then pour them into the bread machine. Then I combine the liquid ingredients (using water at room temperature) and pour them over the dry ingredients in the bread machine.]

2. Set controls and bake.

Per serving

CALORIES: 200 FAT: 4g PROTEIN: 3g CARBOHYDRATES: 40g SODIUM: 224mg CHOLESTEROL: 37mg FIBER: 0.5g

■ ■ ■

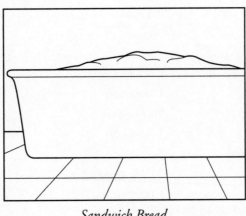

Sandwich Bread

Sopaipillas

Sopaipillas "puff" better if you cut the dough into 3- to 4-inch triangles and gently press the "puffed" portion of the dough into the hot oil as it fries. Serve with honey or powdered sugar.

MAKES 18 SOPAIPILLAS OR 9 SERVINGS

1 tablespoon sugar

1 tablespoon active dry yeast

¾ cup plus 2 tablespoons warm water (110°F)

3 cups flour blend (page 11)

2 teaspoons xanthan gum

½ teaspoon salt

1 teaspoon cider vinegar

1 tablespoon canola oil

1 large egg white

Vegetable oil for frying

1. Dissolve 1 teaspoon of the sugar and the yeast in ¾ cup of the water in a bowl. Let stand for 5 minutes, or until foamy.

2. Combine the flour blend, remaining 2 teaspoons sugar, xanthan gum, and salt in a large mixing bowl. Stir the vinegar into the yeast mixture and add to the dry ingredients with the oil and egg white. Beat with an electric mixer on low speed, adding the remaining 2 tablespoons water until a thick but soft dough forms. Beat the dough on high speed for 1 minute.

3. Cover the bowl and let rise in a warm place (75°F to 80°F) about 1 hour, or until doubled. Roll the dough out to ¼-inch thickness on a work surface that is lightly floured with white rice flour. Cut into 3- to 4-inch triangles.

4. In a deep 3- to 4-quart saucepan, heat 2 to 3 inches of oil to 350°F on a deep-frying thermometer. (An electric fryer works well because the temperature is controlled.)

5. Drop the triangles of dough, flat side down, into the hot oil. When the sopaipilla puffs, gently push the portion where the bubble is developing into the hot oil to help it puff evenly. Cook, turning several times, until pale gold, 1 to 2 minutes total cooking time. With a slotted spoon, transfer the sopaipillas as they are done to paper towels to drain.

Per serving

CALORIES: 205 FAT: 2g PROTEIN: 3g CARBOHYDRATES: 46g
SODIUM: 126mg CHOLESTEROL: 0mg FIBER: 1g

◼ ◼ ◼

Cinnamon Rolls

The heavenly aroma of cinnamon rolls baking in the oven evokes warm memories of home. This recipes makes a nice, light sweet roll drizzled with icing. For the more decadent sticky buns, use your favorite recipe for the topping. These are surprisingly easy to make, so start baking.

MAKES 15 ROLLS

DOUGH

2¼ teaspoons dry yeast

¼ cup sugar

¾ cup warm water (110°F)

1½ cups flour blend (page 11)

1½ cups potato starch

⅓ cup dry milk powder or nondairy milk powder

2 teaspoons xanthan gum

1 teaspoon salt

2 large eggs

¼ cup butter or margarine, at room temperature
(see note, page 23)

1 teaspoon cider vinegar

CINNAMON-SUGAR FILLING

½ cup packed light brown sugar

½ teaspoon cinnamon

POWDERED SUGAR ICING

1 cup powdered sugar

1 tablespoon water

1 tablespoon melted margarine
(see note, page 23)

1. To make the dough: Dissolve the yeast and 2 teaspoons of the sugar in the water. Let stand for 5 minutes, or until foamy.

2. In a large mixer bowl, with an electric mixer on low speed, using regular beaters, not dough hooks, slowly beat the flour blend, potato starch, milk powder, xanthan gum, salt, and the remaining sugar until blended. Reduce speed to low. Add the yeast mixture, eggs, butter, and vinegar; beat just until blended. In-crease speed to high and beat for 2 minutes. Dough will be very sticky. (Use white rice flour during the shaping of the rolls to reduce the stickiness.)

3. Generously grease a 9 x 13-inch non-stick baking pan. To make the filling: Combine the sugar and cinnamon in a small bowl.

4. Divide the dough into 3 equal pieces. Place one piece of dough on a work surface very liberally dusted with rice flour; very generously dust the dough itself with rice flour to prevent sticking. Pat the dough into a ½-inch-thick, 8-inch square, using more rice flour to prevent sticking if necessary. Sprinkle with one-third of the filling. Cut into 5 strips. Roll up each strip and place, cut side up, in prepared pan, pressing dough down lightly to make all rolls a uniform height. Repeat with remaining dough and filling, placing rolls an equal distance apart in 5 rows of 3 rolls each.

5. Cover the rolls and let rise in a warm place (75°F to 80°F) for about 1 hour, or until rolls touch each other and the sides of the pan.

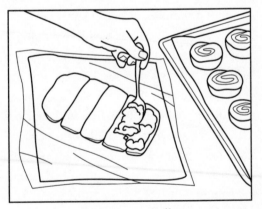

Cinnamon Rolls

6. Preheat the oven to 350°F. Bake the rolls for 20 to 25 minutes, until the tops are nicely browned. Cool in the pan on a wire rack for 10 minutes. Remove the rolls from the pan and cool completely

7. To make the icing: Combine all the ingredients in a small bowl. Drizzle the icing over the rolls. These are best served soon after baking.

Per roll

CALORIES: 245 FAT: 4g PROTEIN: 2g CARBOHYDRATES: 51g SODIUM: 190mg CHOLESTEROL: 30mg FIBER: 0.5g

■ ■ ■

Banana Bread

Don't throw away those extra-ripe bananas! Their high sugar level and fuller flavor makes them perfect for banana bread. If you have too many bananas and aren't ready to bake, just freeze the pulp until you need it.

MAKES 12 SERVINGS

¼ cup canola oil

⅔ cup packed light brown sugar

2 large eggs

1 teaspoon vanilla extract

1¾ cups flour blend (page 11)

2 teaspoons baking powder

1½ teaspoons xanthan gum

½ teaspoon salt

1 teaspoon ground cinnamon

⅛ teaspoon ground cardamom (optional)

⅛ teaspoon ground mace (optional)

1½ cups mashed ripe bananas
   (about 3 medium)

½ cup chopped pecans or walnuts

½ cup raisins

1. Preheat the oven to 350°F. Grease 9 x 5-inch nonstick pan, or for smaller loaves, grease 3 (5 x 3-inch) nonstick pans.

2. Beat the oil and sugar together in a large bowl until creamy. Add the eggs and vanilla and beat well.

3. In a medium bowl, combine the flour blend, baking powder, xanthan gum, salt, cinnamon, and the cardamom and mace, if using. Add the flour mixture to the egg mixture, alternating with the bananas. Stir in the nuts and raisins.

4. Bake the 9 x 5-inch loaf for 1 hour and bake the 5 x 3-inch loaves for 45 minutes, or until a toothpick inserted in the center of the loaf comes out clean. Cool in the pan on a wire rack for 10 minutes. Remove the bread from the pan and cool completely on wire rack before slicing.

Per serving

CALORIES: 170 FAT: 5g PROTEIN: 2g CARBOHYDRATES: 31g SODIUM: 121mg CHOLESTEROL: 23mg FIBER: 1g

■ ■ ■

Boston Brown Bread

Very, very easy to make—a lot like the famous bread from Boston, only you bake this bread rather than steam it.

MAKES 6 SERVINGS

1 ½ cups flour blend (page 11)

¼ cup cornmeal

¼ cup packed light brown sugar

1 teaspoon baking soda

1 teaspoon unflavored gelatin powder

1 ½ teaspoons xanthan gum

¼ teaspoon salt

½ teaspoon ground cinnamon

¼ teaspoon ground allspice

¼ teaspoon ground ginger

¼ teaspoon ground cloves

½ cup raisins

1 cup buttermilk or 1 tablespoon cider vinegar
    plus enough milk (cow, rice, or soy) to equal
    1 cup

1 large egg, lightly beaten

¼ cup molasses

½ teaspoon vanilla extract

2 tablespoons canola oil

1. Preheat the oven to 350°F. Grease 3 (5 x 3-inch) nonstick loaf pans.

2. Combine the flour blend, cornmeal, sugar, baking soda, gelatin, xanthan gum, salt, and spices in a large bowl. Add the raisins and mix well. In another bowl, combine the buttermilk, egg, molasses, vanilla, and oil. Stir the liquid ingredients into the dry ingredients with a spatula until blended. Divide batter equally among prepared pans.

3. Bake for 30 minutes. Remove the bread from the pans and cool on a wire rack.

Per serving

CALORIES: 300 FAT: 5g PROTEIN: 5g CARBOHYDRATES: 63g
SODIUM: 268 mg CHOLESTEROL: 24mg FIBER: 1g

■ ■ ■

Cheese Biscotti

Part cracker, part bread—this biscotti is a variation of the traditional sweet biscotti. Serve these crisp, cheese-flavored sticks with soups or salads. They travel very well; I've even taken them to Europe.

MAKES 24 BISCOTTI OR 8 SERVINGS

2 cups flour blend (page 11)

¼ teaspoon salt

1 teaspoon xanthan gum

1 teaspoon baking powder

2 tablespoons sugar

1 teaspoon dried rosemary

½ cup gluten-free light sour cream or sour
    cream alternative

2 tablespoons olive oil

¼ cup corn syrup

3 large egg whites

½ cup shredded Swiss or Cheddar cheese
(cow or soy)

2 teaspoons grated Parmesan cheese (cow or
soy), plus additional for dusting (optional)

1½ cups sunflower seeds

2 teaspoons dried chives

1. Preheat the oven to 350°F. Grease a 13 x 9-inch nonstick baking sheet or line with parchment paper.

2. In a food processor, combine the flour blend, salt, xanthan gum, baking powder, sugar, and rosemary. Process with on/off pulses until mixed.

3. Lightly beat together the sour cream, oil, corn syrup, egg whites, and cheeses in another bowl. Pour the egg-white mixture evenly over the dry ingredients in the food processor and pulse on and off about twenty times to moisten dough. Add the sunflower seeds and chives and pulse to incorporate.

4. Form the dough into a ball, divide in half, and shape each half into a 2-inch wide, ½-inch-thick, 12-inch-long log. Arrange on the prepared baking sheet.

5. Bake for 20 minutes, or until the logs brown at the edges. Cool on wire rack for 5 minutes. Leave the oven on.

6. With sharp knife (an electric knife works well), cut each log diagonally into ¾-inch-thick slices. Arrange slices, cut side down, on the baking sheet and return them to the oven.

7. Bake for 5 to 7 minutes, until the biscotti start to brown. Transfer to a wire rack to cool. Dust with additional Parmesan, if desired.

Per serving
CALORIES: 135 FAT: 5g PROTEIN: 3g CARBOHYDRATES: 22g SODIUM: 64mg CHOLESTEROL: 3mg FIBER: 1g

■ ■ ■

Corn Bread

Corn bread is one of the ultimate comfort foods. I like to serve it with Mexican or southwestern meals because its mild, earthy flavor complements spicy foods. This version is very easy to assemble, and the recipe is very forgiving. For a crispy crust, bake it in a preheated cast-iron skillet. Grease it carefully (so you don't burn yourself) just before you pour in the corn bread batter.

MAKES 12 SERVINGS

1¼ cups cornmeal

1 cup flour blend (page 11)

⅓ cup sugar

2 teaspoons baking powder

1½ teaspoons xanthan gum

1 teaspoon salt

2 large eggs

1 cup milk (cow, rice, or soy)

⅓ cup canola oil

1. Preheat the oven to 350°F. Grease an 8-inch-round or -square nonstick pan or a preheated cast-iron skillet; set aside.

2. In a medium bowl, combine the cornmeal, flour blend, sugar, baking powder, xanthan gum, and salt and beat with an electric mixer on low speed just until blended. Add the eggs, milk, and oil. Increase speed to medium and beat until well blended. The batter will be the consistency of thick cake batter.

3. Transfer the batter to the prepared pan. Bake for 25 to 30 minutes, until top is firm and edges are lightly browned. Serve warm.

Per serving
CALORIES: 185 FAT: 8g PROTEIN: 3g CARBOHYDRATES: 26g CHOLESTEROL: 33mg SODIUM: 340mg FIBER: 1g

■ ■ ■

Corn Tortillas

Okay, I know you buy corn tortillas in the grocery store. But, if you've ever tasted a homemade corn tortilla, you know there is no comparison. These are absolutely wonderful! These tortillas are especially easy to make with a tortilla press (under twenty dollars in kitchenware departments).

MAKES 12 TORTILLAS; 6 SERVINGS

2 cups corn flour (*not* cornmeal)
1¼ cups warm water

1. In a food processor, blend corn flour and water until it forms a smooth ball. Divide the dough into 12 equal pieces and shape into balls. Cover to prevent dough from drying out.

2. Cut 24 pieces of waxed paper, each about 7 inches square. Place one square of waxed paper on the bottom half of the tortilla press. Place a ball of dough slightly off center toward the edge opposite the handle. Place another piece of waxed paper on top of the dough. Lower the top of the tortilla press and press down firmly on the handle. This makes a tortilla that is 6 to 6½ inches in diameter. Remove the tortilla, keeping it between the waxed paper, and stack on a plate. Repeat with remaining dough.

3. To fry, heat a griddle or electric skillet on high heat until hot. Holding a tortilla in your left hand, peel off the top layer of waxed paper with your right hand, starting with the side nearest your left wrist and pulling the paper up toward the ceiling. Carefully invert the tortilla onto the griddle. Wait 3 seconds; peel off the remaining waxed paper. Do not leave the waxed paper on the tortilla for longer than 3 seconds because it will permanently cook into the tortilla.

4. Cook the tortilla about 2 minutes on each side, until it looks dry and has golden flecks on it. Transfer the tortilla to a plate to cool, stacking them between sheets of waxed

paper. Repeat with remaining tortillas. Refrigerate in a resealable plastic bag. Reheat to serve.

Per serving

CALORIES: 140 FAT: 2g PROTEIN: 3g CARBOHYDRATES: 30g SODIUM: 8mg CHOLESTEROL: 0mg FIBER 5g

■ ■ ■

Flour Tortillas

This is a Santa Fe tortilla, which is thicker and somewhat less pliable than the purchased kind. Tortillas are best when freshly made and warm from the grill.

MAKES 4 TORTILLAS

½ teaspoon soy lecithin granules

½ teaspoon honey

½ cup boiling water

¼ cup evaporated skim milk or nondairy milk
   minus 1 tablespoon

1½ teaspoons canola oil

1 cup brown rice flour

½ cup potato starch

¼ cup arrowroot

1 teaspoon salt

1 teaspoon cream of tartar

½ teaspoon baking soda

1. Stir the lecithin and honey into the water in a medium bowl until the lecithin has dissolved. Cool 10 minutes. Add the milk and oil.

2. Meanwhile, sift the rice flour, potato starch, arrowroot, salt, cream of tartar, and baking soda into a food processor. Add the liquid mixture and process until a soft ball is formed. Cut the dough into 4 pieces and shape into balls. Cover tightly and refrigerate for 2 hours.

3. Between heavily floured sheets of waxed paper or plastic wrap, roll each ball into a 7- to 8-inch circle, adding rice flour to prevent sticking. Remove the waxed paper. In an electric skillet on high heat, cook each tortilla on both sides until brown speckles form. Wrap in foil immediately. Serve warm.

Per tortilla

CALORIES: 265 FAT: 32g PROTEIN: 5g CARBOHYDRATES: 53g SODIUM: 643mg CHOLESTEROL: 1mg FIBER: 0.5g

■ ■ ■

Popovers

The secret to successful popovers is to get the baking pan piping hot before adding the batter and baking the popovers at a very high temperature. A special popover pan (with narrower and deeper molds) also helps, but you can use your traditional 6-cup muffin pan or custard cups.

MAKES 6 POPOVERS

3 eggs, at room temperature

¾ cup milk (cow, soy, rice), at room temperature

1 tablespoon canola oil

⅔ cup potato starch

¼ cup flour blend (page 11)

½ teaspoon salt

¼ teaspoon xanthan gum

1. Preheat the oven to 450°F. Place a 6-cup nonstick muffin pan or 6 custard cups in the oven while it is preheating.

2. Combine the eggs, milk, and oil in a blender and blend thoroughly. Add the potato starch, flour blend, salt, and xanthan gum and blend until thoroughly mixed.

3. Just before pouring the batter into the pan, remove it from the oven and spray with cooking spray, then dust with rice flour. Fill each cup about half full with batter. Bake for 20 minutes at 450°F, then reduce the temperature to 350°F and bake for 15 minutes, or until the sides of the popovers are rigid to the touch. Do not open the oven until the popovers are done because this may cause them to collapse. Serve warm.

Per popover

CALORIES: 180 FAT: 5g PROTEIN: 5g CARBOHYDRATES: 29 SODIUM: 229mg CHOLESTEROL: 121mg FIBER: 1g

VARIATION

Yorkshire Pudding

Pour 1 teaspoon of hot meat drippings into each cup. Add popover batter and bake as directed.

Per serving

CALORIES: 190 FAT: 6g PROTEIN: 5g CARBOHYDRATES: 29g SODIUM: 233mg CHOLESTEROL: 122mg FIBER: 0.5g

Note: For high-altitude baking, increase the number of eggs to four.

■ ■ ■

Scones

Even though scones can be served at afternoon tea, this version is more rustic and hearty for eating anytime.

MAKES 6 SCONES

1¼ cups brown rice flour or sorghum flour

½ cup tapioca flour

1 ½ teaspoons cream of tartar

¾ teaspoon baking soda

1 ½ teaspoons xanthan gum

¼ teaspoon salt

¼ cup sugar

¼ cup butter or margarine (see note, page 23), chilled and cut into ½-inch pieces

1 large egg, lightly beaten

⅔ cup plain yogurt or ½ cup nondairy milk

⅓ cup currants

2 tablespoons milk (cow, soy, rice), for brushing

1. Preheat the oven to 450°F. Grease a baking sheet or line with parchment paper.

2. In a food processor, combine the flours, cream of tartar, baking soda, xanthan gum, salt, and sugar; pulse on and off until mixed. Add the butter and pulse about 15 to 20 times, until the mixture resembles coarse meal.

3. Combine the egg and yogurt in a small bowl. Pour over the dry ingredients and process for about 10 seconds, or until large curds form. Add the currants and pulse a few times to incorporate. Remove dough from the food processor and shape it into a ball.

4. On the prepared baking sheet, pat the dough out to a ¾-inch-thick, 8-inch circle. Brush the top with the milk. Bake for 12 to 15 minutes, until browned, firm, and slightly crusty on the surface. Cut into 6 wedges.

Per scone

CALORIES: 260 FAT: 7g PROTEIN: 4g CARBOHYDRATES: 50g SODIUM: 266mg CHOLESTEROL: 39mg FIBER: 1g

■ ■ ■

Crackers

These great crackers travel well and can be frozen. The rounder you can make each cracker, the more professional they will look.

MAKES ABOUT 20 CRACKERS

¼ cup garbanzo/fava bean flour or sorghum flour

¼ cup potato starch

¼ cup sweet rice flour

½ teaspoon xanthan gum

¼ teaspoon baking soda

½ teaspoon salt, plus additional for sprinkling (optional)

½ teaspoon onion powder

2 tablespoons grated Parmesan cheese (cow or soy)

2 tablespoons butter or margarine (see note, page 23), at room temperature

1 tablespoon honey or pure maple syrup

3 tablespoons toasted sesame seeds, plus additional for sprinkling (optional)

2 tablespoons milk (cow, rice, soy, or nut)

1 teaspoon cider vinegar

1. Preheat the oven to 350°F. Grease a baking sheet or line with parchment paper.

2. In a food processor, combine all the ingredients and process until the mixture forms a ball.

3. Shape the dough into 20 (1-inch) balls, and place at least 2 inches apart on the prepared baking sheet. Using the bottom of a drinking glass or rolling pin, flatten the balls to about ⅛-inch thickness. With your fingers, smooth the edges of the crackers.

4. Bake for 12 to 15 minutes, until the crackers look firm and slightly toasted. Turn each cracker and bake 5 to 7 minutes longer, until golden brown. Sprinkle with additional sesame seeds and salt, if desired.

Per Cracker

CALORIES: 50 FAT: 2 g PROTEIN: 1g CARBOHYDRATES: 7g SODIUM: 93 mg CHOLESTEROL: 1 mg FIBER: 0.5g

■ ■ ■

Pretzels

Pretzels make great snacks and travel very well. Make them thin and crispy for easy munching or make them thick and chewy for more serious consumption. Store them in airtight containers.

MAKES 30 PRETZELS

1 tablespoon dry yeast

½ teaspoon sugar

⅔ cup warm water (110°F)

½ cup sorghum flour

½ cup tapioca flour

1 tablespoon dry milk powder or nondairy
   milk powder

2 teaspoons xanthan gum

1 teaspoon onion powder

1 teaspoon unflavored gelatin powder

½ teaspoon salt

1 tablespoon olive oil

1 teaspoon cider vinegar

1 large egg white, beaten until foamy

1 tablespoon coarse salt, or to taste

1. Dissolve the yeast and sugar in the water in a small bowl. Let stand for 5 minutes, or until foamy.

2. In a medium bowl, with a mixer on low speed, blend the flours, milk powder, xanthan gum, onion powder, gelatin, and salt. Add the yeast mixture, oil, and vinegar. Increase speed to high; beat for 3 minutes.

3. Cut a diagonal ¼-inch opening on one corner (this makes a ½-inch circle) of a large, heavy-duty, resealable plastic freezer bag and place the dough in the bag. Squeeze the dough out of the plastic bag onto the prepared baking sheet. Straight 3-inch sticks are easiest to make. For the best results, hold the bag of dough upright as you squeeze, rather than at an angle, and position the seam of the bag on top, instead of at the side. Brush the strips lightly with the egg white, then sprinkle with the coarse salt. Let the pretzels rise in a warm place (75°F to 80°F) for 10 to 15 minutes.

4. Preheat the oven to 400°F. Bake for 15 minutes, or until the pretzels are dry and golden brown. Transfer the pretzels to a wire rack to cool completely. Store in an airtight container.

Per pretzel

CALORIES: 25 FAT: 0.5g PROTEIN: 1g CARBOHYDRATES: 4g SODIUM: 227mg CHOLESTEROL: 0mg FIBER: 0.5g

VARIATION

For softer, chewier pretzels increase the cut in the plastic bag to ⅓ inch (this makes a ⅔-inch circle). Follow the recipe above, but let the pretzels rise for 5 to 10 minutes longer or until they reach the size you want. Remember, they'll rise more as they bake. Bake as directed above, but remove from the oven when they're nicely browned, but before they become dry and crisp.

■ ■ ■

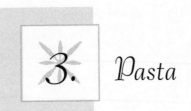

3. Pasta

Who can imagine spaghetti and meatballs without the spaghetti? Or macaroni and cheese without the macaroni? Pasta is definitely one of the foods we miss the most on a gluten-free diet.

With today's abundance of wonderful, gluten-free pastas, there's no reason to go without. Although there are many good brands available, I find myself reaching for the Pastariso and DeBole's at the health food store, or ordering Dr. Shar's penne pasta, which I discovered in Tuscany a few years ago, or Bi-Aglut from the many gluten-free vendors listed in the Mail-Order Sources (page 257).

There are still some folks who prefer to make their own pasta and, I must admit, there's something really special about fresh, homemade pasta. So, for the purists who insist on fresh pasta, you'll find a wonderfully easy recipe that's sure to please.

I heartily recommend that you invest in an electric pasta machine; it will save you countless hours. But you can also make delicious noodles, fettuccine, and lasagne by hand and never need anything but a sharp knife and a little patience.

When you're cooking pasta, use plenty of water—about one quart for each pound of pasta. If you don't use enough water, you may end up with a sticky blob. Here's why: As the pasta cooks, various starches dissolve in the water. Our gluten-free pasta is a bit starchier than regular pasta because of a lower protein content. If there's plenty of water in the pot, the starches don't cause a problem. However, if there's not enough water in the pot, the starches form a sticky, starchy tangle. Keeping the water at a strong boil so that the bubbles in the water move the pasta around will also help keep the dissolved starches and pasta from sticking.

You'll often see the words *al dente* in relation to cooking pasta. They literally mean "to the tooth" and indicate that the pasta should be not quite done when you remove it from the boiling water. In addition, pasta continues to cook after it's removed from the boiling water, so you need to factor that into the allotted cooking time.

Homemade Egg Pasta

This pasta is absolutely heavenly, easy to make, and freezes well. If despite the proliferation of wonderful commercial gluten-free pasta, you still like to make your own, this recipe is for you!

MAKES 4 SERVINGS; 4 CUPS, CUT
INTO NOODLES

2 large eggs

¼ cup water

1 tablespoon canola oil for hand method or
   1 teaspoon for electric pasta machine

½ cup brown rice or sorghum flour

½ cup tapioca flour

½ cup cornstarch

¼ cup potato starch

4 teaspoons xanthan gum

1 teaspoon unflavored gelatin powder

½ teaspoon salt

To make by hand:

1. Combine the eggs, water, and oil in a food processor and process until the eggs are light yellow in color. Add the remaining ingredients; process until thoroughly blended and mixture forms a ball. Remove the cover of the food processor and break up the dough into smaller egg-sized pieces. Replace the cover and process until a ball forms again.

2. Transfer the dough to a pastry board or smooth surface. Roll dough between two sheets of waxed paper or plastic wrap dusted with rice flour. Roll as thinly as possible and cut into desired shapes with a sharp knife or pastry cutter. Cook in boiling water until still firm but tender to the bite, about 5 minutes.

To make in an electric pasta machine:

Follow the manufacturer's instructions, because different machines require different processes. My machine calls for first placing 1 teaspoon oil in the machine and thoroughly mixing together and adding the dry ingredients. Combine the eggs and water; whisk together until light yellow and foamy, breaking up all egg membranes thoroughly before slowly adding the mixture to the machine. Withhold 2 tablespoons of the egg mixture until you're sure it's needed. Mix as directed.

Per serving
CALORIES: 290 FAT: 6g PROTEIN: 8g CARBOHYDRATES: 49g SODIUM: 303mg CHOL: 106mg; FIBER: 0.5g

VARIATIONS

Basil-Garlic Pasta
Add 1 teaspoon dried basil and ½ teaspoon garlic powder.

Spinach Pasta
Cook 1 cup packed fresh spinach leaves in boiling water for 5 minutes. (Or use ½ cup frozen spinach, thawed). Drain all but 2 tablespoons of water from the spinach. Using a handheld blender, purée the spinach until smooth. Use puréed spinach mixture in place of the ¼ cup water.

Tomato Pasta
Substitute ¼ cup tomato juice for the ¼ cup water.

Chile Pasta
Add 1 teaspoon New Mexico chile powder.

Note: The fresh pasta can be dried either by hanging on a pasta drying rack or it can be separated and dried on baking sheets. Store the dried pasta in the freezer.

■ ■ ■

Ravioli

Although ravioli takes a little time to make, it is well worth the effort. Be sure to avoid getting filling or oil on the edges of the ravioli, or they won't form a seal.

MAKES ABOUT 30 RAVIOLI; 4 SERVINGS

Homemade Egg Pasta (page 49)
1 tablespoon *each* shredded mozzarella and grated Romano cheese or nondairy cheese of choice
½ cup ricotta cheese or firm silken tofu, creamed
1 teaspoon Italian seasoning
1 large egg, separated
1 tablespoon water
1½ cups Spaghetti Sauce (page 88)
½ cup grated Parmesan cheese (cow or soy), for garnish

1. Prepare the pasta dough. In a small bowl, combine the mozzarella, Romano, and ricotta cheeses, Italian seasoning, and egg yolk; set aside.

2. Beat the egg white and water in a small bowl until smooth; set aside.

3. Roll out the pasta dough to about a 12-inch square on a potato starch–floured surface. Brush half of the dough with the egg-white mixture. Place teaspoonfuls of the cheese mixture about 2 inches apart on the egg-painted side of the dough. Fold the unpainted half of the dough over the cheese mounds and seal the edges with your fingers. Press the dough between the mounds together with your fingers.

4. With a pastry cutter, cut the ravioli into squares where you've pressed the dough together, or use a special pastry tool that both cuts and crimps dough at the same time.

5. Cook the ravioli in boiling, salted water for 5 to 10 minutes, until just tender. Drain. Serve with the sauce and garnish with the Parmesan cheese.

Per serving

CALORIES: 305 FAT: 15g PROTEIN: 14g CARBOHYDRATES: 29g SODIUM: 795mg CHOLESTEROL: 107mg FIBER: 3g

■ ■ ■

Fettuccine Alfredo

This is fabulous. It has a lower fat content than the traditional version, but it is still a decadent dish in terms of fat and calories. Unfortunately for those with dairy sensitivities, it is dairy based.

MAKES 4 SERVINGS

1½ cups cottage cheese

3 tablespoons skim milk (cow, rice, or soy)

¼ cup grated Parmesan cheese

1 small garlic clove, minced

2 tablespoons butter

Homemade Egg Pasta (page 49), cut into noodles, or 4 cups purchased gluten-free fettuccine, cooked

¼ cup chopped fresh parsley

1 teaspoon lemon pepper

1. In a food processor, combine the cottage cheese, milk, Parmesan, garlic, and butter; process until the mixture is very, very smooth.

2. Transfer the mixture to a medium heavy saucepan and whisk over medium heat until it reaches serving temperature.

3. Pour mixture over hot cooked pasta. Garnish with the parsley and lemon pepper.

Per serving

CALORIES: 800 FAT: 23g PROTEIN: 31g CARBOHYDRATES: 114g SODIUM: 1,178mg CHOLESTEROL: 232mg FIBER: 2g

■ ■ ■

Linguine with Pine Nuts

This is quick, easy, and delicious. It makes a great dish for company.

MAKES 4 SERVINGS

½ recipe Homemade Egg Pasta (page 49), cut
    into linguine, or 2 cups purchased gluten-free
    linguine pasta
½ teaspoon salt
¼ cup pine nuts
¼ cup chopped fresh parsley, plus additional
    for garnish
¼ cup grated Parmesan cheese (cow or soy)
1 teaspoon lemon pepper
2 tablespoons olive oil

1. Add pasta and salt to pot of boiling water. Cook pasta until still firm but tender to the bite, about 5 minutes for fresh pasta.

2. While the pasta cooks, toast the pine nuts in a preheated 350°F oven for 5 to 10 minutes or in a dry skillet over medium heat 5 to 10 minutes, until lightly browned. Watch carefully so that they don't burn.

3. Drain the pasta and toss with remaining ingredients. Garnish with parsley. Serve immediately.

Per serving
CALORIES: 420 FAT: 15g PROTEIN: 13g CARBOHYDRATES: 58g SODIUM: 785mg CHOLESTEROL: 106mg FIBER: 1g

Pasta with Lemon and Herbs

This dish boasts a delicate lemon flavor that marries well with the herb seasoning.

MAKES 4 SERVINGS

Homemade Egg Pasta (page 49), cut into
    noodles, or 4 cups purchased gluten-free
    penne pasta, cooked
2 tablespoons olive oil
1 tablespoon dried chives
1 tablespoon dried parsley
¼ teaspoon black pepper
2 tablespoons fresh lemon juice
1 teaspoon grated lemon zest
½ teaspoon herb seasoning (such as fines
    herbes)
4 tablespoons grated Parmesan cheese
    (cow or soy)

1. Combine the hot pasta with the remaining ingredients, using 3 tablespoons of the Parmesan, and toss gently to combine. Garnish with the remaining Parmesan. Serve warm.

Per serving
CALORIES: 730 FAT: 22g PROTEIN: 20g CARBOHYDRATES: 111g SODIUM: 770mg CHOLESTEROL: 208m FIBER: 2g

Macaroni and Cheese

This is the ultimate comfort food: smooth, creamy, and so satisfying. Because of the cheese, this dish is dairy based, but you can try using nondairy cheese. Just remember, nondairy cheese won't melt as well, look as shiny, or be as smooth as regular cheeses.

MAKES 6 SERVINGS

1 teaspoon cornstarch or arrowroot

1 teaspoon salt

¼ teaspoon cayenne pepper

2½ cups skim milk (cow, rice, or soy)

1 tablespoon Dijonnaise mustard

1 cup shredded extra-sharp Cheddar cheese

½ cup mozzarella cheese

½ cup plus 1 tablespoon grated Parmesan
    cheese (cow or soy)

10 ounces purchased gluten-free elbow
    macaroni, cooked

1. In a heavy ovenproof skillet or pan, combine the cornstarch, salt, cayenne, and milk; mix well. Bring to a boil and boil, stirring constantly, for 1 minute. Stir in the mustard, Cheddar, mozzarella, and the ½ cup Parmesan.

2. Preheat the broiler. Stir the macaroni into the cheese sauce. Sprinkle with the remaining 1 tablespoon Parmesan and broil until the top is browned.

Per serving
CALORIES: 345 FAT: 9g PROTEIN: 20g CARBOHYDRATES: 44g SODIUM: 725mg CHOLESTEROL: 27mg FIBER: 1g

■ ■ ■

Pasta Salad Primavera

Primavera means "spring" in Italian, and this combination of pasta and springtime vegetables is delightful. You can vary the vegetables as you wish. Add chopped chicken or cooked shrimp for an entrée,

MAKES 4 SERVINGS

1 cup diagonally sliced asparagus

1 cup diagonally halved snow peas

1 tablespoon plus 1 teaspoon olive oil

¼ cup chopped onion

½ recipe Homemade Egg Pasta (page 49), cut
    into noodles, or 2 cups purchased gluten-free
    penne pasta

2 tablespoons dry white wine

1 tablespoon balsamic vinegar

½ teaspoon salt

¼ teaspoon white pepper

1 garlic clove, minced

½ cup grated Parmesan cheese (cow or soy),
    plus additional for garnish

½ cup chopped red bell pepper

¼ cup chopped fresh parsley

1. Cook the asparagus and snow peas in boiling water in a large saucepan for 1 to 2 minutes. Plunge immediately into ice water to prevent further cooking. Set aside.

2. Heat 1 tablespoon oil in a small skillet over medium-low heat. Add the onion and sauté until tender, about 5 minutes. Set aside.

3. In boiling water, cook the pasta until slightly al dente, about 5 minutes. Drain thoroughly and transfer to a large bowl. Add the wine, vinegar, the remaining 1 teaspoon oil, salt, white pepper, garlic, Parmesan, bell pepper, and parsley, and toss until the pasta is evenly coated.

4. Add the asparagus, snow peas, and onion; toss until thoroughly combined. Garnish with Parmesan.

Per serving

CALORIES: 765 FAT: 21g PROTEIN: 23g CARBOHYDRATES: 117g SODIUM: 1257mg CHOLESTEROL: 212mg FIBER: 3g

■ ■ ■

Italian Pasta Salad

The black olives and basil give this tasty side dish an Italian flair. You can vary the vegetables as you wish. Add chopped chicken or Italian cold cuts (most Boar's Head brand deli meats are gluten-free) to make an entrée.

MAKES 4 SERVINGS

2 tablespoons olive oil

¼ cup chopped onion

½ recipe Homemade Egg Pasta (page 49), cut into wide noodles, or 2 cups purchased gluten-free penne pasta

1 cup broccoli florets

1 tablespoon Dijonnaise mustard

1 tablespoon balsamic vinegar

2 tablespoons cider vinegar

2 tablespoons fresh lemon juice

1 garlic clove, minced

½ cup chopped red bell pepper

½ cup black olives

¼ cup chopped fresh basil

¼ teaspoon black pepper

½ cup grated Parmesan cheese (cow or soy)

1. Heat 1 tablespoon of the oil in a small skillet over medium heat. Add the onion and sauté until tender. Set aside.

2. Cook the pasta in a pot of boiling water until slightly al dente, about 5 minutes, adding the broccoli during the last minute of cooking. Drain well. Plunge the broccoli into ice water to prevent further cooking.

3. Transfer the pasta and broccoli to a bowl. Add the mustard, vinegars, and lemon juice. Add the sautéed onion, remaining 1 tablespoon oil, garlic, bell pepper, olives, basil, black pepper, and Parmesan. Toss gently but thoroughly. Cover and refrigerate until chilled for flavors to blend. Let stand at room temperature for 20 minutes before serving.

Per serving

CALORIES: 765 FAT: 23g PROTEIN: 24g CARBOHYDRATES: 116g SODIUM: 1,117 mg CHOLESTEROL: 248mg FIBER: 3g

■ ■ ■

Greek Pasta Salad

This is a wonderful summer salad. Add cooked chicken or salmon if you want to serve it as a main dish. Feta cheese is usually made from goat's milk or cow's milk; if you have milk allergies you should avoid this dish or omit the feta.

MAKES 4 SERVINGS

DRESSING

¼ cup red wine vinegar

¼ cup fresh lemon juice

2 tablespoons dry white wine

¼ teaspoon sugar

¼ teaspoon salt

¼ teaspoon white pepper

¼ cup olive oil

SALAD

2 cups purchased gluten-free rotini or
   penne pasta

⅓ cup ½-inch pieces yellow bell pepper

⅓ cup ½-inch pieces red bell pepper

¼ cup ¼-inch pieces green onion tops

⅓ cup chopped dry-pack sun-dried tomatoes

⅓ cup pitted black olives, halved

½ cup crumbled feta cheese

⅓ cup pine nuts, toasted (see page 52)

1 small garlic clove, minced

1. To make the dressing: In a screw-top jar, combine the vinegar, lemon juice, wine, sugar, salt, and pepper. Shake vigorously until the sugar has dissolved. Add the oil and shake again. Set aside.

2. To make the salad: Cook the pasta in boiling water until slightly al dente. Drain thoroughly and transfer to a large bowl.

3. Add the dressing to the pasta and toss to combine. Add the remaining ingredients and toss to combine.

4. Refrigerate the salad until chilled to blend the flavors. Let stand at room temperature for 20 minutes before serving.

Per serving

CALORIES: 450 FAT: 24g PROTEIN: 12g CARBOHYDRATES: 48g SODIUM: 490mg CHOLESTEROL: 13mg FIBER: 3g

■ ■ ■

Mediterranean Pasta Salad

This salad evokes images of warm sunny beaches and the clear blue skies of the Mediterranean. It makes a very colorful salad and can be combined with cooked chicken or salmon for a heartier main dish.

MAKES 4 SERVINGS

DRESSING

1/4 cup red wine vinegar

2 tablespoons fresh lemon juice

1 teaspoon Dijonnaise mustard

1/4 teaspoon salt

1/4 teaspoon white pepper

1/4 cup olive oil

SALAD

1 cup broccoli florets

1 cup snow peas

2 cups purchased gluten-free rotini or
   penne pasta

1 tablespoon dried basil

1 small garlic clove, minced

1 small red bell pepper, chopped

1/4 cup pitted Kalamata olives, halved

1/4 cup pine nuts, toasted (see page 52)

1. To make the dressing: In a screw-top jar, combine the vinegar, lemon juice, mustard, salt, pepper, and olive oil. Shake vigorously to blend. Set aside.

2. To make the salad: Cook the broccoli and snow peas in boiling water in a large saucepan for 1 to 2 minutes. Plunge immediately into ice water to prevent further cooking. Set aside.

3. Cook the pasta in boiling water until slightly al dente. Drain thoroughly and transfer to a large bowl. Immediately add the dressing and toss to combine.

4. Add the remaining ingredients to the pasta; toss thoroughly. Refrigerate until chilled to blend the flavors. Let stand at room temperature for 20 minutes before serving.

Per serving

CALORIES: 540 FAT: 26g PROTEIN: 13g CARBOHYDRATES: 66g SODIUM: 730mg CHOLESTEROL: 102mg FIBER: 4g

■ ■ ■

Asian Soba Noodles

Pure buckwheat soba noodles are made by Eden Foods. Don't mistakenly buy the kind that contains wheat. Despite its name, buckwheat is not actually wheat (or grain) but rather the fruit of a plant related to rhubarb. You may substitute gluten-free spaghetti if pure buckwheat noodles are not available or if you don't like buckwheat. This dish is delicious served with grilled fish.

MAKES 6 SERVINGS

1 pound pure buckwheat soba noodles

1/4 teaspoon salt

2 tablespoons sesame oil

2 tablespoons water

1/4 cup low-sodium, wheat-free tamari soy sauce

2 tablespoons sugar or honey

1 1/2 tablespoons red wine vinegar

1 cup chopped fresh cilantro

1/2 cup chopped green onions

½ jalapeño chile, chopped

½ cup diced red bell pepper

½ cup pine nuts, toasted (see page 52)

1. Cook the noodles in a large pot of rapidly boiling water with the salt for about 10 minutes, or until just tender. Drain and immerse the noodles in ice water until cool. Drain well. Transfer to a large bowl.

2. Combine the sesame oil, water, soy sauce, sugar, and vinegar in a screw-top jar. Shake the dressing vigorously until the sugar has dissolved; pour over the noodles. Add the cilantro, green onions, chile, and bell pepper; mix well. Sprinkle the pine nuts over the salad and serve.

Per serving

CALORIES: 430 FAT: 16g PROTEIN: 17g CARBOHYDRATES: 66g SODIUM: 1,014mg CHOLESTEROL: 0mg FIBER: 1g

■ ■ ■

4. Grains & Beans

This chapter focuses on the wonderful side dishes that complement our meals and provide an important source of carbohydrates, the energy food. Included here are recipes for beans and grains—dishes that often use wheat as a thickener or binder. I emphasize grains in this chapter because they're chock-full of nutrients, and they provide important fiber, especially when they're consumed in their natural, unrefined state.

What's for Breakfast? And Lunch? And Dinner?

Cooked grains are an essential and very nutritious component of a healthy, gluten-free diet. For example, hot cereal is an absolute necessity at breakfast for many of us. Just because you don't eat wheat doesn't mean you can't have cooked cereal.

At lunch and dinner, hot cooked grains become interesting, nutritious side dishes, especially when joined by flavorful herbs, toasted nuts, and sautéed vegetables.

How to Cook Whole Grains

Although many of these alternative grains are used in the recipes in this chapter, the following table gives you basic guidelines on how to cook them. Use salt as you wish. One cup of grain makes four servings.

GRAIN (1 CUP)	WATER	COOKING TIME
Amaranth	2 cups	15 to 20 minutes
Brown rice	2½ cups	30 to 45 minutes
Buckwheat	1 cup	15 to 20 minutes
Corn grits	3 cups	5 minutes
Millet	3½ to 4 cups	35 to 45 minutes
Quinoa (KEEN-wah)	2 cups	15 to 20 minutes
White rice	2 cups	15 to 20 minutes
Wild rice	4 cups	40 minutes

Mexican Rice

This lightly spiced rice dish is perfect with a Mexican or southwestern meal.

MAKES 4 SERVINGS

1 teaspoon canola oil

1 cup chopped onion

1 garlic clove, minced

1 cup long-grain white rice

1 cup low-sodium, gluten-free chicken broth

½ teaspoon dried oregano

1 (10-ounce) can tomatoes with green chiles
(such as Rotel's), undrained

½ cup chopped fresh cilantro

¼ cup sliced black olives

Heat the oil in a large saucepan over medium heat. Add the onion and sauté, stirring frequently, for 3 to 5 minutes. Add the garlic, rice, broth, oregano, and tomatoes with juice; bring to a boil. Reduce heat and simmer, covered, for 20 to 25 minutes, until the liquid has been absorbed. Stir in the cilantro and olives and serve.

Per serving
CALORIES: 220 FAT: 3g PROTEIN: 7g CARBOHYDRATES: 44g SODIUM: 490mg CHOLESTEROL: 0mg FIBER: 1g

■ ■ ■

Herbed Brown Rice

You can use chicken, beef, or vegetable broth in this dish. Dried herbs work better than fresh in this recipe because fresh herbs will overwhelm the color of the dish and turn it very green.

MAKES 6 SERVINGS

1 tablespoon olive oil

1 cup chopped onion

1 (12-ounce) package long-grain brown rice

2 garlic cloves, minced

1½ cups low-sodium, gluten-free chicken broth

1 teaspoon *each* dried basil, chives, and parsley

¾ teaspoon black pepper

½ teaspoon salt

1. Preheat the oven to 350°F. Heat the oil in a 3-quart, ovenproof saucepan over medium heat. Add the onion and sauté, stirring frequently, for 5 minutes. Add the rice; cook, stirring, for 2 minutes. Stir in the remaining ingredients.

2. Cover and transfer to the oven. Bake for 40 minutes, or until the rice is tender.

Per serving
CALORIES: 240 FAT: 4g PROTEIN: 7g CARBOHYDRATES: 47g SODIUM: 388mg CHOLESTEROL: 0mg FIBER: 1g

■ ■ ■

Curried Rice Pilaf with Raisins

Basmati rice is a fragrant, aromatic rice originally grown in India and Pakistan. It is a favorite for pilafs because of its nutty flavor.

MAKES 4 SERVINGS

1 tablespoon peanut oil

1 cup chopped onion

1½ teaspoons curry powder

1 teaspoon chile powder

1 cup basmati or long-grain white rice

½ cup golden raisins

½ teaspoon salt

2 cups low-sodium, gluten-free chicken broth

½ cup sliced almonds, toasted (see page 63)

1. Heat the oil in a large heavy saucepan over medium heat. Add the onion, curry powder, and chile powder and sauté, stirring frequently, for about 5 minutes, or until the onion is tender. Stir in the rice, raisins, and salt.

2. Add the broth; cover and simmer for about 20 minutes, or until the broth has been absorbed and the rice is tender. Sprinkle with the almonds just before serving.

──────────

Per serving

CALORIES: 380 FAT: 14g PROTEIN: 14g CARBOHYDRATES: 59g SODIUM: 685mg CHOLESTEROL: 0mg FIBER: 3g

■ ■ ■

Quinoa, Wild Rice, and Cranberry Pilaf

Quinoa is an ancient grain from the Incas in Peru and one of the most nutritious grains on earth. You can substitute dried cherries for the cranberries, if you like.

MAKES 6 SERVINGS

¾ cup wild rice, rinsed

3 cups low-sodium, gluten-free chicken broth

½ cup whole-grain quinoa

¼ cup dried cranberries

¼ cup golden raisins

1 teaspoon olive oil

⅓ cup sliced almonds, toasted (see page 63)

1. In a saucepan, combine the rice and broth and bring to a boil. Reduce the heat, cover, and simmer for 15 minutes.

2. Meanwhile, preheat the oven to 325°F. Rinse the quinoa in a sieve, rubbing the grains between your fingers. Drain and repeat until the water runs clear, two or three times.

3. Remove the rice from the heat. Stir in the quinoa, cranberries, raisins, and oil. Spoon the mixture into a 1½-quart greased casserole. Bake, covered, for 1 hour, or until the rice and quinoa are tender and the liquid has been absorbed. Sprinkle with the almonds.

──────────

Per serving

CALORIES: 235 FAT: 7g PROTEIN: 12 g CARBOHYDRATES: 33g SODIUM: 789mg CHOLESTEROL: 1mg FIBER: 3g

■ ■ ■

Rice Pilaf with Dried Fruits and Nuts

This is a very flavorful rice pilaf, packed with lots of texture from the dried fruits and nuts. It makes a wonderful dish for company and goes well with pork or chicken.

MAKES 6 SERVINGS

¼ teaspoon ground cloves

⅛ teaspoon ground saffron

⅛ teaspoon ground allspice

1 tablespoon butter

½ cup chopped onion

1 garlic clove, minced

½ teaspoon salt

1 cup long-grain white rice

2 cups low-sodium, gluten-free chicken broth

½ cup chopped dried apricots

½ cup golden raisins

½ cup dried cherries

½ cup sliced almonds, toasted (see page 63)

1 tablespoon chopped fresh parsley

1. Combine the spices and set aside.

2. Melt the butter in a large, heavy pan over medium heat. Add the onion and garlic and sauté, stirring frequently, until the onion is limp. Add the spice mixture and salt and cook, stirring constantly, for 1 minute, until the spices are slightly toasted.

3. Stir in the rice and cook for 1 minute. Add the broth, apricots, raisins, and cherries and cook, covered, for about 20 minutes, until the liquid has been absorbed or until the rice is tender. Stir in the almonds; sprinkle with the parsley.

Per serving

CALORIES: 330 FAT: 10g PROTEIN: 10mg CARBOHYDRATES: 55g SODIUM: 778mg CHOLESTEROL: 7mg FIBER: 3g

■ ■ ■

Risotto with Mushrooms and Herbs

The creamy texture and delicate flavor of this risotto are very palate pleasing. Be sure to use arborio rice so the end result will be more like traditional risotto.

MAKES 4 SERVINGS

1½ tablespoons extra-virgin olive oil

1 small onion, finely chopped

1 garlic clove, minced

1½ cups arborio or medium-grain rice

4 cups low-sodium, gluten-free chicken broth

½ cup dry white wine

1 teaspoon dried basil leaves

1 teaspoon dried thyme leaves

1 teaspoon dried rosemary

1 tablespoon fresh or 1 teaspoon dried chives

$\frac{1}{2}$ pound fresh mushrooms, sliced

4 tablespoons grated Parmesan cheese
   (cow or soy)

$\frac{1}{2}$ teaspoon salt

$\frac{1}{4}$ teaspoon white pepper

1. Heat the oil in large, heavy saucepan over medium heat. Add the onion and garlic and sauté, stirring frequently, for about 5 minutes, until the onion is soft but not brown. Stir in the rice and cook, stirring constantly, for about 1 minute, until all the grains are shiny.

2. Heat the broth in a saucepan over medium heat until hot. Adjust the heat to keep it hot but not boiling.

3. Add the wine to the rice and bring to a boil, stirring constantly. When most of the wine has been absorbed, add $\frac{1}{2}$ cup of the hot broth. Cook the rice, stirring constantly, at a gentle boil. When most of liquid has been absorbed, add another $\frac{1}{2}$ cup broth. Continue adding the broth, $\frac{1}{2}$ cup at a time and stirring constantly, until all the broth is used. If the rice seems hard, add another $\frac{1}{2}$ cup of hot broth or water

4. Remove the pan from the heat and stir in the herbs, mushrooms, Parmesan, salt, and pepper. Serve hot.

Per serving

CALORIES: 390 FAT: 8g PROTEIN: 20g CARBOHYDRATES: 64g SODIUM: 1,024mg CHOLESTEROL: 4mg FIBER: 3g

■ ■ ■

Saffron Rice Pilaf

Saffron gives this dish a delicate flavor and color. It goes especially well with fish.

MAKES 4 SERVINGS

2 tablespoons slivered almonds

1 teaspoon canola oil

1 onion, finely chopped

2 tablespoons pine nuts

1 cup long-grain white rice

$2\frac{1}{4}$ cups low-sodium, gluten-free chicken broth

$\frac{1}{4}$ teaspoon ground saffron

2 teaspoons grated lemon zest

$\frac{1}{2}$ cup golden raisins

$\frac{1}{2}$ teaspoon salt

$\frac{1}{2}$ teaspoon dried thyme leaves

$\frac{1}{8}$ teaspoon ground cardamom

1 tablespoon chopped fresh parsley

1. Toast the almonds in a pie plate in a 400°F oven for 5 minutes, or until golden brown. Set aside.

2. Heat the oil in a medium heavy saucepan over medium heat. Add the onion and pine nuts and sauté, stirring frequently, 5 to 7 minutes, until the onion is soft and the pine nuts are lightly browned.

3. Stir in the rice and cook, stirring frequently, 3 to 4 minutes. (This lightly toasts the rice and produces a richer flavor.) Add the

broth, saffron, lemon zest, raisins, salt, thyme, and cardamom; stir well. Reduce the heat to low, cover, and simmer for 15 to 20 minutes, until all the liquid has been absorbed.

4. Remove the pan from the heat and fluff the rice with a fork. Stir in the almonds and sprinkle with the parsley. Serve hot.

Per serving
CALORIES: 205 FAT: 4g PROTEIN: 9g CARBOHYDRATES: 38g SODIUM: 468mg CHOLESTEROL: 0mg FIBER: 3g

■ ■ ■

Wild Rice Pancakes with Pecans

Pancakes make an unusual but very delectable side dish for an elegant dinner. You can serve them plain or with a topping such as applesauce, sour cream, chives, or your favorite sauce or gravy.

MAKES 12 PANCAKES; 4 SERVINGS

⅔ cup wild rice, rinsed

3 cups low-sodium, gluten-free chicken broth

½ cup brown rice flour

½ teaspoon baking powder

½ teaspoon baking soda

¼ teaspon ground black pepper

2 tablespoons dried chives

¼ teaspoon dried thyme

½ teaspoon salt

1 large egg

½ cup buttermilk or 1 teaspoon cider vinegar with enough milk (cow, rice, or soy) to equal ½ cup

¼ cup chopped pecans

1 tablespoon canola oil

1. Combine the rice and broth in a medium, heavy saucepan over medium heat and bring to a boil. Reduce the heat, cover, and simmer for about 40 minutes, until the rice is tender, or the liquid has been absorbed. Drain. Cool to room temperature.

2. Mix the rice flour, baking powder, baking soda, pepper, chives, thyme, and salt in a medium bowl.

3. In a small bowl, whisk together the egg and buttermilk. Add to the flour mixture and stir until well blended. Mix in the cooked rice and pecans.

4. Lightly coat a large nonstick skillet over medium heat with the oil; heat until hot. Drop the batter by tablespoonfuls onto the skillet to form 3-inch pancakes, cooking in batches if necessary. Cook for about 2 minutes per side, until golden brown. Repeat with the remaining batter, using more oil if necessary.

Per serving
CALORIES: 225 FAT: 5g PROTEIN: 16g CARBOHYDRATES: 35g SODIUM: 908mg CHOLESTEROL: 46mg FIBER: 2g

■ ■ ■

Wild Rice with Dried Fruit

The combination of nutty, crunchy wild rice and the sweet yet tart flavor of dried fruit makes an irresistible dish. It especially complements roast pork or roast chicken.

MAKES 4 SERVINGS

1 cup wild rice, rinsed

$\frac{1}{2}$ cup chopped green onions

3 cups water

$\frac{1}{2}$ cup diced dried apricots

$\frac{1}{4}$ cup golden raisins

2 tablespoons chopped fresh parsley

$\frac{1}{4}$ cup pine nuts, toasted (see page 52)

1 teaspoon olive oil

2 tablespoons balsamic vinegar

2 tablespoons fresh orange juice

$\frac{1}{4}$ teaspoon grated orange zest

1 garlic clove, minced

$\frac{1}{4}$ teaspoon salt

$\frac{1}{8}$ teaspoon ground black pepper

1. Combine the rice, green onions, and water in a medium heavy saucepan over medium heat and bring to a boil. Reduce the heat to low, cover, and simmer for 45 minutes, until tender, or until liquid has been absorbed. Drain.

2. Transfer the rice to a large bowl. Stir in the apricots, raisins, parsley, and pine nuts. Toss gently to combine.

3. Combine the oil, vinegar, orange juice, orange zest, garlic, salt, and pepper in a screw-top jar. Shake vigorously to blend well. Pour dressing over rice mixture and toss gently. Serve hot.

Per serving

CALORIES: 270 FAT: 6g PROTEIN: 9g CARBOHYDRATES: 50g SODIUM: 150mg CHOLESTEROL: 0mg FIBER: 5g

■ ■ ■

Tabbouleh

This dish is a delicious variation of the traditional tabbouleh made with bulgur wheat. You'll never miss the wheat. Go easy with the feta cheese; a little goes a long way. Avoid it if you're dairy sensitive.

MAKES 4 SERVINGS

1 cup whole-grain quinoa or 1 cup long-grain brown rice

$\frac{3}{4}$ teaspoon salt

2 cups water

$\frac{1}{4}$ cup shelled pumpkin seeds or pine nuts

2 tablespoons fresh lemon juice

3 tablespoons olive oil

1 tablespoon wine vinegar

$\frac{1}{8}$ teaspoon ground white pepper

1 cucumber, chopped

3 green onions, chopped

1 large red bell pepper, diced

½ cup chopped fresh parsley

½ cup chopped fresh cilantro

¼ cup chopped fresh mint

¼ cup crumbled feta cheese (optional)

1. Rinse the quinoa in a sieve, rubbing the grains between your fingers. Drain and repeat until the water runs clear, two or three times. Transfer the quinoa to a large heavy skillet and toast over medium heat for about 4 minutes, until light golden brown.

2. In a medium heavy saucepan, combine the quinoa (or brown rice), ½ teaspoon of the salt, and water; bring to a boil. Cover, reduce the heat, and simmer for 12 to 15 minutes, until tender. Transfer the quinoa to a strainer and drain well.

3. Meanwhile, toast the pumpkin seeds in a skillet over medium heat, stirring constantly, for about 5 minutes, until lightly browned.

4. Combine the lemon juice, oil, vinegar, remaining ¼ teaspoon salt, and white pepper in a screw-top jar. Shake vigorously to blend.

5. Combine the quinoa and all of the remaining ingredients, including the dressing, in a large bowl; toss well. Cover and refrigerate for 4 hours for flavors to blend. Let stand at room temperature for 20 minutes before serving.

Per serving

CALORIES: 370 FAT: 16g PROTEIN: 13g CARBOHYDRATES: 50g SODIUM: 556 CHOLESTEROL: 6mg FIBER: 7g

▪ ▪ ▪

Polenta with Mushrooms

A traditional Italian dish, polenta has been revived and has even gained "gourmet" status in many restaurants. This version is very easy, and the mushrooms add an interesting texture. I use regular cornmeal, although there is a coarser version, sometimes called corn grits, especially for polenta. Of course, you can always buy ready-made polenta, but my motto is "Fresh is always better."

MAKES 4 SIDE-DISH SERVINGS

1 tablespoon olive oil

1 small onion, chopped

3 tablespoons water

2 cups chopped fresh mushrooms
   (shiitake, button, or crimini)

1 tablespoon butter or margarine
   (see note, page 23)

½ teaspoon dried oregano

¾ teaspoon salt

⅛ teaspoon ground black pepper

¾ cup low-sodium, gluten-free chicken broth

1 cup milk (cow, rice, or soy)

½ cup water

½ cup regular cornmeal

2 tablespoons grated Parmesan cheese
   (cow or soy)

1. Heat the oil in a 12-inch skillet over medium heat. Add the onion and water and

cook until the onion is tender and lightly browned. With a slotted spoon, transfer the onion to a plate and set aside.

2. To the same skillet, add the mushrooms, butter, oregano, ¼ teaspoon of the salt, and the pepper and cook, stirring constantly, for 3 to 5 minutes. Add ¼ cup of the broth and boil for 1 minute to thicken slightly. Remove from the heat and keep warm.

3. In a large saucepan over high heat, combine the milk, remaining ½ teaspoon salt, and remaining ½ cup broth and bring to a boil. Reduce the heat to low. Gradually sprinkle in the cornmeal, whisking constantly, and cook, stirring constantly, for 5 minutes, or until thick. Stir in the Parmesan cheese and reserved onion. Serve the polenta topped with the mushroom mixture.

Per serving

CALORIES: 150 FAT: 5g PROTEIN: 8g CARBOHYDRATES: 20g SODIUM: 713mg CHOLESTEROL: 4mg FIBER: 2g

■ ■ ■

Boston Baked Beans

No picnic is complete without this summer favorite.

MAKES 10 SERVINGS

2 cups dried navy beans, picked over and rinsed
4 cups water
½ cup dark molasses
¼ cup packed light brown sugar

1 teaspoon dry mustard (see note, page 68)
¼ teaspoon ground cloves
¼ teaspoon chile powder
¼ teaspoon black pepper
2 tablespoons instant chopped onion
⅓ cup ketchup
½ teaspoon salt

1. Place the beans in a large Dutch oven. Add enough water to cover the beans by 2 inches and bring to a boil. Remove from the heat and let stand overnight. Drain the beans and return them to the Dutch oven.

2. Preheat the oven to 325°F. Combine the beans with the 4 cups water and the remaining ingredients, except the ketchup and salt. Cover and bake, stirring occasionally, for 3½ to 4 hours. Stir in the ketchup and salt, recover, and bake for 30 to 45 minutes, until the beans are tender. (Don't add the salt any sooner; it may toughen the beans.)

Per serving

CALORIES: 215 FAT: 0.5g PROTEIN: 10g CARBOHYDRATES: 45g SODIUM: 213mg CHOLESTEROL: 0mg FIBER: 10g

VARIATION

If you don't have time for this long-simmering version, substitute 2 (about 16 ounces each) cans of rinsed and drained pork and beans for the dried navy beans. Combine all the remaining ingredients (except water) in a microwave-safe dish. Heat to serving temperature in the microwave.

Note: If you can't find Durkee or Spice Islands dry mustard, you can grind your own mustard seeds with a small coffee grinder. Some preground dry mustard contains wheat.

■ ■ ■

Southwestern Beans

Beans are a staple in the Southwest. Here, they're combined with interesting herbs and spices to produce a wonderful blend of flavors and aromas.

MAKES 6 SERVINGS

1 slice bacon

1 small onion, chopped

1 garlic clove, minced

1 bay leaf

2 teaspoons dried oregano

1 teaspoon ground cumin

1/8 teaspoon ground cloves

1 teaspoon gluten-free instant
  coffee powder

1 tablespoon light brown sugar

1 pound dried pinto beans, picked
  over and rinsed

6 cups water

Salt, to taste

1. In a heavy Dutch oven, fry the bacon until crisp and brown. Transfer the bacon to paper towels to drain. When cool, crumble the bacon.

2. Add the onion to the bacon drippings and sauté over medium heat, stirring occasionally, until golden brown. Return the crumbled bacon to the pan and add the remaining ingredients; bring to a boil. Reduce the heat, cover, and cook for 2 to 3 hours, until the beans are tender. Season with salt.

Per serving
CALORIES: 330 FAT: 6g PROTEIN: 19g CARBOHYDRATES: 52g SODIUM: 265mg CHOLESTEROL: 8mg FIBER: 19g

VARIATIONS

Slow Cooker
After combining all the ingredients in step 2, transfer the mixture to a slow cooker and cook on medium-high heat for 2 to 3 hours, depending on temperature settings of slow cooker.

Refried Beans
To fry beans, place 1 teaspoon canola oil in a large, heavy skillet that has been sprayed with cooking spray. Add 2 cups cooked Southwestern Beans. Mash beans completely, using a potato masher or spatula. Cook, uncovered, over medium heat, stirring often, for about 10 minutes, until thick.

■ ■ ■

Red Beans and Rice

If you're fond of Cajun food, the spicy, flavorful cuisine found in certain parts of the Southeast, you'll love this dish. It's high in fiber and low in fat and calories, but it's sure to satisfy your quest for flavor.

MAKES 6 SERVINGS

1 teaspoon olive oil

1 small yellow onion, chopped

1 celery stalk, chopped

3 garlic cloves, minced

1 pound dried small red beans (not kidney beans), picked over and rinsed

1 smoked ham hock, well trimmed and cut into thick slices

1 teaspoon dried basil

1 teaspoon dried tarragon

1 teaspoon dried rosemary

2 bay leaves

1½ teaspoons salt

1 teaspoon ground black pepper

⅓ cup packed light brown sugar

2 dashes hot pepper sauce

4 cups cooked white rice

1 tablespoon chopped fresh parsley

1. Heat the oil in a large heavy saucepan over medium heat. Add the onion, celery, and garlic and sauté, stirring frequently, until the onion is translucent.

2. Combine the beans, ham hock, herbs, bay leaves, salt, pepper, brown sugar, and hot pepper sauce in a large saucepan. Add enough water to cover the beans and bring to a boil. Boil for 10 minutes. Reduce the heat, cover, and simmer over medium heat for 2 hours, or until the beans are tender. Discard the bay leaves. Serve over the rice. Garnish with the parsley.

Per serving

CALORIES: 400 FAT: 2g PROTEIN: 17g CARBOHYDRATES: 80g SODIUM: 557mg CHOLESTEROL: 0mg FIBER: 15g

VARIATION

Slow Cooker
Combine all of the ingredients in a slow cooker and cook on low heat all day, about 8 hours.

◼ ◼ ◼

Lentil Tabbouleh

This nontraditional version of tabbouleh uses lentils instead of bulgur wheat. The lentils provide a hefty dose of fiber. If you add chopped chicken or pork, you'll have a hearty main dish.

MAKES 4 SERVINGS

4 cups water

1 cup brown lentils

1 garlic clove, peeled

1 bay leaf

1/2 teaspoon salt

1/2 teaspoon ground black pepper

1 cucumber, peeled and chopped

1 small red bell pepper, diced

1/4 cup chopped red onion

1/2 cup chopped fresh mint

1/2 cup chopped fresh parsley

1 teaspoon fresh lemon juice

1 teaspoon fresh lime juice

2 teaspoons red wine vinegar

1 1/2 tablespoons olive oil

1. In a large saucepan, combine the water, lentils, garlic, bay leaf, salt, and pepper. Bring to a boil over medium heat. Reduce the heat to low, cover, and simmer for about 30 minutes, until the lentils are tender. Drain the lentils and discard the bay leaf and garlic. Transfer the lentils to a large bowl and set aside to cool.

2. Add the cucumber, bell pepper, onion, mint, and parsley to the lentils.

3. In a screw-top jar, combine the lemon juice, lime juice, vinegar, and oil; shake vigorously until well blended. Pour the dressing over the lentil mixture and gently toss to combine. Cover and refrigerate for 4 hours or overnight. Serve chilled or at room temperature.

───────────

Per serving

CALORIES: 235 FAT: 6g PROTEIN: 15g CARBOHYDRATES: 34g SODIUM: 285mg CHOLESTEROL: 0mg FIBER: 16g

■ ■ ■

Veggieburgers

Gluten-free vegetarians will enjoy this hearty, meatless burger. You'll never miss the meat! Substitute 1 1/3 cups cooked garbanzo beans for the quinoa, if you prefer.

MAKES 16 PATTIES; 8 SERVINGS

2/3 cup whole grain quinoa

3 cups water

2/3 cup brown lentils

2/3 cup long-grain brown rice

1/4 cup canola or olive oil, plus additional for frying

2 cups grated carrots

1 cup chopped onion

1 cup chopped celery

1/4 cup shelled sunflower seeds

1 large garlic clove, minced

1 teaspoon dried basil

1 teaspoon dried thyme

1 teaspoon dried oregano

1 teaspoon salt

1/2 teaspoon ground black pepper

2 tablespoons Dijonnaise mustard

4 large eggs, lightly beaten

6 tablespoons brown rice flour

Hamburger Buns (page 26), optional

Lettuce leaves and sliced tomatoes (optional)

Condiments

1. Rinse the quinoa in a sieve, rubbing the grains between your fingers. Drain and repeat two or three times, until the water runs clear. Drain.

2. Bring the water to a boil in a medium heavy saucepan over high heat. Add the quinoa, lentils, and rice. Cover and reduce the heat to low. Cook for about 40 minutes, until the grains are tender. Drain and cool.

3. Heat the oil in a heavy skillet over medium-low heat. Add the carrots, onion, celery, sunflower seeds, and garlic and sauté, stirring occasionally, for 8 to 10 minutes. Cool slightly. Add to the grains.

4. Add the herbs, salt, and pepper to the grains. Transfer 1 cup of the mixture to a food processor and purée. Return the purée to the grain mixture.

5. Stir the mustard, eggs, and rice flour into the grain mixture. With your hands, form ½ cupfuls of the mixture into patties.

6. Heat a little oil in a heavy skillet over medium heat until hot. Add the patties and cook for about 5 minutes per side, until golden brown.

7. Serve the patties plain or on Hamburger Buns, if you prefer. Garnish with lettuce, tomatoes, and condiments of choice, if you like.

Per serving (burgers only)
CALORIES: 320 FAT: 12g PROTEIN: 12g CARBOHYDRATES: 43g SODIUM: 325mg CHOLESTEROL: 90mg FIBER: 8g

■ ■ ■

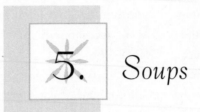

5. *Soups*

Soups can be a low-fat, low-calorie component of a flavorful, highly nutritious diet. People on a gluten-free diet, however, sometimes avoid soups for several reasons. Wheat is often used as the thickener, especially in cream soups, or the bouillon base used in the soup may contain gluten. Often a small amount of wheat-based pasta is included in the recipe, making the entire soup off-limits.

Of course, there are many soups that are safe for gluten-sensitive people. You'll find them in any cookbook. For this reason, the recipes in this chapter are those that usually contain gluten, but I've converted them to gluten-free versions so you and I can enjoy them.

Cheese Soup

Hearty and flavorful, all you need with this soup is crusty French Bread (page 25) and you have a robust meal. This recipe is dairy based and works better with dairy rather than soy Cheddar cheese.

MAKES 5 TO 6 CUPS; 4 SERVINGS

2 tablespoons canola oil

¼ cup finely chopped onion

⅓ cup sweet rice flour

3 cups low-sodium, gluten-free chicken broth

½ teaspoon dry mustard (see note, page 68)

½ teaspoon paprika

⅛ teaspoon cayenne pepper

½ teaspoon salt

1 cup skim milk

1½ cups shredded extra-sharp Cheddar cheese

¼ cup minced fresh chives or 2 tablespoons dried chives

1. Heat the oil in a large Dutch oven over medium heat. Add the onion and sauté until soft.

2. In a screw-top jar, combine the flour and 1 cup of the broth. Shake vigorously to blend well. Add the flour mixture, the remaining broth, and the remaining ingredients, except the cheese and chives, to the Dutch oven. Cook over medium heat, stirring constantly, until the mixture comes to a boil and thick-ens. Reduce the heat to low, add the cheese, and cook, stirring, until the cheese has melted and the soup is smooth.

3. To serve, ladle the soup into 4 soup bowls. Garnish with chives.

Per serving
CALORIES: 300 FAT: 21g PROTEIN: 20g CARBOHYDRATES: 13g SODIUM: 860mg CHOLESTEROL: 46mg FIBER: 0.5g

■ ■ ■

Cream of Broccoli Soup

The combination of basil and broccoli gives this rich and creamy soup a delightful flavor.

MAKES 4 SERVINGS

3 cups broccoli florets

1 cup low-sodium, gluten-free chicken broth

1 teaspoon olive oil

1 cup chopped onion

1 garlic clove, minced

1½ tablespoons cornstarch or 3 tablespoons sweet rice flour

2 cups evaporated skim milk or 1¾ cups milk (cow, rice, or soy)

½ teaspoon salt

¼ teaspoon ground white pepper

1½ teaspoons dried basil

⅛ teaspoon ground nutmeg

1. Coarsely chop the broccoli and place in a medium saucepan. Add the broth and boil for about 5 minutes, until fork-tender. Set aside to cool, but don't drain.

2. Heat the oil in a heavy skillet over medium heat. Add the onion and garlic and sauté for 8 to 10 minutes, until tender.

3. Combine the cornstarch with ¼ cup of the broth used to cook the broccoli in a small bowl; stir to form a smooth paste. Add the remaining broth to the skillet. Stir in the cornstarch mixture and cook over medium-low heat, whisking constantly, until the mixture thickens.

4. Add the broccoli with broth, the milk, salt, pepper, basil, and nutmeg. Heat to serving temperature, but do not boil.

Per serving

CALORIES: 180 FAT: 2g PROTEIN: 16g CARBOHYDRATES: 28g SODIUM: 296mg CHOLESTEROL: 5mg FIBER: 4g

■ ■ ■

Cream of Mushroom Soup

The rich flavor of mushrooms is tantalizing. Canned mushrooms work better because they don't turn dark. If you prefer to buy your mushroom soup, Progresso cream of mushroom soup is gluten-free.

MAKES 4 SERVINGS

1 teaspoon olive oil

1 cup chopped onion

1 garlic clove, minced

3 cups evaporated skim milk or soy or rice milk

1½ tablespoons cornstarch or 3 tablespoons sweet rice flour mixed with ¼ cup water

3 (7-ounce) cans (3 cups) sliced or chopped mushrooms, drained

½ teaspoon salt

¼ teaspoon ground white pepper

1½ teaspoons dried parsley

⅛ teaspoon ground nutmeg

½ teaspoon dried thyme

1. Heat the oil in a large heavy saucepan over medium heat. Add the onion and garlic and sauté for 8 to 10 minutes, until the onion is tender.

2. Stir in the milk and heat until bubbles form around the edges. Stir the cornstarch mixture until blended. Whisk the cornstarch mixture into the milk mixture and cook, whisking constantly, until the mixture thickens slightly, but do not boil.

3. Stir in the mushrooms and remaining ingredients. Heat to serving temperature, but do not boil.

Per serving

CALORIES: 155 FAT: 2g PROTEIN: 14g CARBOHYDRATES: 25g SODIUM: 280mg CHOLESTEROL: 5mg FIBER: 2g

■ ■ ■

French Onion Soup

This soup derives its deep flavor from the caramelized onions that take nearly an hour to cook, but it's worth the effort! Instead of Gruyère or Swiss cheese, you can use your favorite nondairy version; however, it won't melt as smoothly.

MAKES 4 SERVINGS

3 tablespoons olive oil

1 tablespoon butter or margarine (see note, page 23)

2 pounds onions, sliced

½ teaspoon salt

½ teaspoon ground black pepper

½ teaspoon sugar

2 garlic cloves, minced

4 cups low-sodium, gluten-free beef broth

1 cup water

2 teaspoons brandy extract

¼ teaspoon dried marjoram leaves

1 bay leaf

1 tablespoon sweet rice flour mixed with
  1 tablespoon water

½ loaf French Bread (page 25)

2 cups shredded Gruyère or Swiss cheese or nondairy cheese of choice

2 tablespoons grated Parmesan cheese (cow or soy), for garnish

1. Heat the oil and butter in a heavy Dutch oven over medium heat. Add the onions, salt, and pepper; cook, stirring occasionally, for about 10 minutes, or until the onions begin to soften. Reduce the heat to low and cook slowly, stirring occasionally, for about 1 hour and 15 minutes, until the onions are caramelized. (After 30 minutes of cooking, the onions should be light golden brown. After another 45 minutes, the onions will be deep brown, the secret of good French onion soup.)

2. Slowly stir the sugar, garlic, broth, water, brandy extract, marjoram, and bay leaf into the onions. Simmer, partially covered, for 15 minutes. Stir the flour mixture, add to the soup, and cook, stirring constantly, until slightly thickened.

3. Meanwhile, preheat the oven to 325°F. Cut the bread crosswise into ¾-inch-thick slices. Arrange the bread slices in a single layer on a baking sheet and bake 5 minutes per side, or until dry.

4. Preheat the broiler. Ladle the soup into heatproof soup bowls. Place a slice of toasted bread on top of the soup in each bowl. Divide the Gruyère cheese equally among the bowls. Broil for 2 to 3 minutes, until golden brown. Garnish with the Parmesan cheese.

Per serving

CALORIES: 605 FAT: 33g PROTEIN: 35g CARBOHYDRATES: 42mg SODIUM: 2,238mg CHOLESTEROL: 71mg FIBER: 5g

VARIATION

Southwestern French Onion Soup

Instead of the thyme, use ½ teaspoon toasted ground cumin, ¼ teaspoon ground coriander, ¼ teaspoon dried oregano, and 1 tablespoon New Mexico ground red chile powder. Instead of Gruyère or Swiss cheese, substitute Monterey Jack cheese with jalapeño chiles. Garnish with 2 tablespoons fresh chopped cilantro.

Per serving

CALORIES: 585 FAT: 32g PROTEIN: 33g CARBOHYDRATES: 42g SODIUM: 2,350mg CHOLESTEROL: 59mg FIBER: 5g

■ ■ ■

Minestrone

If you don't have gluten-free pasta on hand, you can omit it in this classic Italian soup, but it does lend a nice flair.

MAKES 4 SERVINGS

1 cup *each* coarsely chopped carrots
   and cabbage
4 cups low-sodium, gluten-free beef broth
½ cup dry white navy beans, picked over
   and rinsed
2 garlic cloves, minced
½ cup chopped onion
1 cup diced potatoes
1 cup canned tomatoes
¼ cup green beans
¼ teaspoon red pepper flakes
½ teaspoon *each* dried basil, thyme, sage,
   and oregano
¼ teaspoon salt
1 cup fresh spinach, coarsely chopped
¼ cup purchased gluten-free elbow macaroni
¼ cup grated Parmesan cheese (cow or soy),
   for garnish

1. In a large heavy Dutch oven, combine all the ingredients, except the spinach, pasta, and Parmesan cheese, and bring to a boil. Reduce the heat, cover, and simmer for at least 3 hours or until the beans are tender.

2. Stir in the spinach and pasta; cook just until the pasta is tender. Garnish with Parmesan cheese.

Per serving

CALORIES: 210 FAT: 3g PROTEIN: 22g CARBOHYDRATES: 36g SODIUM: 909mg CHOLESTROL: 17mg FIBER: 9g

■ ■ ■

Chicken Noodle Soup

*E*veryone loves comforting chicken noodle soup. This version is flavor-packed with herbs and spices. If you prefer a simpler version, reduce the seasonings. Add the dumplings, and you have a really hearty soup—perfect for a cold winter's night.

MAKES 4 SERVINGS

3 cups low-sodium, gluten-free chicken broth

1/2 cup thinly sliced celery

1 cup diced cooked chicken

1/4 cup instant chopped onions

1 small carrot, peeled and thinly sliced

1/2 teaspoon poultry seasoning

6 whole peppercorns

1/4 teaspoon ground white pepper

1/8 teaspoon ground nutmeg

1 bay leaf

1/2 cup purchased gluten-free pasta
    (rotini, elbow, or penne)

1 recipe Dumplings (below), optional

1/4 cup chopped fresh parsley

1. Combine all the ingredients, except the pasta, dumplings, and parsley, in a large Dutch oven and bring to a boil over medium heat. Reduce the heat, cover, and simmer for 10 minutes.

2. While the soup simmers, assemble the ingredients for the dumplings, if using, and cook according to recipe directions in a separate pan of water.

3. Add the pasta to the soup and cook for about 5 minutes, or until the pasta is tender. Don't overcook.

4. To serve, divide the soup equally among 4 serving bowls. Add dumplings, if using, and garnish with the parsley.

Per serving

CALORIES: 435 FAT: 12g PROTEIN: 34g CARBOHYDRATES: 55g SODIUM: 844mg CHOLESTEROL: 116mg FIBER: 5g

◾ ◾ ◾

Dumplings

This recipe can be made into big, hearty dumplings for noodle soups or tiny German spaetzle, which are sometimes served with green beans.

MAKES 4 SERVINGS

1 1/4 cups brown rice flour or sorghum flour

2/3 cup potato starch

2 teaspoons baking powder

1/2 teaspoon baking soda

1/2 teaspoon potato flour (*not* potato starch)

1/2 teaspoon salt

1 large egg

3 tablespoons margarine (see note, page 23),
    at room temperature

1/2 cup buttermilk or 1 teaspoon cider vinegar
    plus enough milk (cow, rice, or soy) to
    equal 1/2 cup

2 tablespoons chopped fresh parsley

1. Combine the dry ingredients in a large bowl. Make a well in the center.

2. In another bowl, whisk together the egg and margarine. Alternately add the egg mix-

ture and the buttermilk to the dry ingredients. Stir in the parsley. Mix only until moistened; the dough will be stiff.

3. Drop the dough by tablespoonfuls into boiling water. Cover, reduce the heat to low, and simmer gently for 20 minutes without lifting the lid. Add to soup just before serving.

___

Per serving

CALORIES: 365 FAT: 11g PROTEIN: 8g CARBOHYDRATES: 58g SODIUM: 750mg CHOLESTEROL: 46mg FIBER: 1g

VARIATION

Spaetzle
Add an additional ¼ cup buttermilk when making the dough. To form, press the dough through the holes in a colander or a spaetzle maker into boiling water (or soup). Cook for 1 to 2 minutes, or until the spaetzle float to the top.

■ ■ ■

New England Clam Chowder

Chowders make wonderful lunch dishes. However, teamed up with a hearty bread and a lettuce salad, this soup could be served for supper.

MAKES 4 SERVINGS

1 bacon slice
1 cup chopped onion
½ cup chopped celery
2 garlic cloves, minced
1 (8-ounce) bottle clam broth
1½ cups chopped potatoes
¼ teaspoon salt
⅛ teaspoon ground black pepper
½ teaspoon Beau Monde seasoning or gluten-free seasoning salt
2 tablespoons potato starch
2 cups milk (cow, rice, or soy)
1 cup fresh or 1 (6.5-ounce) can clams with liquid
2 tablespoons chopped fresh parsley

1. Sauté the bacon until crisp in a large Dutch oven at medium heat. With a slotted spoon transfer the bacon to paper towels to drain. Set aside and crumble when cool. Add the onion, celery, and garlic to the bacon drippings and sauté until the vegetables are soft. Return the crumbled bacon to the Dutch oven.

2. Add the clam broth, potatoes, salt, pepper, and Beau Monde seasoning; bring to a boil. Reduce the heat, cover, and simmer for 20 minutes, or until the potatoes are tender.

3. In a small bowl or cup, combine the potato starch and ¼ cup of the milk; stir until smooth. Add the starch mixture to the Dutch oven along with remaining milk and cook, stirring constantly, until the mixture thickens slightly. Stir in the clams. Heat to serving tem-

perature; do not boil. Ladle into 4 serving bowls. Garnish with the parsley.

_____

Per serving
CALORIES: 230 FAT: 12g PROTEIN: 16g CARBOHYDRATES: 16g SODIUM: 618mg CHOLESTEROL: 43mg FIBER: 1g

■ ■ ■

Potato Soup

Potato soup is so comforting! This version makes a great lunch dish or a light Sunday night supper.

MAKES 4 SERVINGS

½ cup low-sodium, gluten-free chicken broth

2 potatoes, peeled and thinly sliced

¼ cup instant chopped onions

½ cup thinly sliced celery

1 small carrot, peeled and grated

½ teaspoon celery salt

3 cups milk (cow, rice, or soy)

½ teaspoon dried marjoram leaves

¼ teaspoon dried thyme leaves

¼ cup chopped fresh parsley

1. Combine the broth, potatoes, onions, celery, carrot, and celery salt in a large nonreactive saucepan; bring to a boil over medium heat. Reduce the heat, cover, and simmer for 10 minutes, or until the potatoes are tender. (Add water if vegetables look dry during cooking.)

2. Remove ½ cup of the potato mixture and purée in a blender or with a handheld immersion blender. Be careful; the mixture is hot. Return the mixture to the pan. Add the milk, marjoram, and thyme and heat to serving temperature, but do not boil.

3. To serve, pour soup into 4 serving bowls. Garnish with the parsley.

_____

Per serving
CALORIES: 160 FAT: 6g PROTEIN: 9g CARBOHYDRATES: 19g SODIUM: 412 mg CHOLESTEROL: 25mg FIBER: 2g

■ ■ ■

Wild Rice Soup

This is a rich-tasting, very satisfying soup with lots of interesting texture.

MAKES 6 SERVINGS

2 tablespoons butter or margarine
   (see note, page 23)

1 tablespoon diced onion

⅓ cup sweet rice flour

3 cups low-sodium, gluten-free chicken broth

2 cups cooked wild rice

½ teaspoon salt

⅓ cup shredded carrot

⅓ cup diced ham or Canadian-style bacon

3 tablespoons slivered almonds, toasted
   (see page 63)

1 cup evaporated skim milk (or rice or soy milk)

¼ cup chopped fresh chives or 2 tablespoons
  dried chives

1. Melt the butter in a large Dutch oven over medium heat. Add the onion and sauté until golden brown.

2. Combine the rice flour and 1 cup of the broth in a screw-top jar. Shake vigorously to blend well. Add to the Dutch oven with the remaining 2 cups broth and bring to a boil. Boil, stirring constantly, for 1 minute. Add the rice, salt, carrot, ham, and almonds and simmer for 5 minutes. Blend in the milk. Heat to serving temperature, but do not boil. Garnish with the chives.

Per serving
CALORIES: 340 FAT: 7g PROTEIN: 19g CARBOHYDRATES: 53g SODIUM: 633mg CHOLESTEROL: 16mg FIBER: 4g

■ ■ ■

6. Sauces & Salad Dressings

I can't imagine food without sauces or salad dressings. All too often, though, gluten-sensitive people avoid sauces or salad dressings because some of the ingredients, usually the thickeners or binders, are unknown. This can leave food bland, boring, and unappealing, but it doesn't have to be that way.

The recipes for sauces and salad dressings in this chapter serve an important role in diets devoid of wheat and gluten. They provide variety in the form of pleasing tastes, interesting textures, and tempting aromas. We all know that when food tastes good and smells good, it is far more satisfying.

Sauces not only add variety in terms of taste, texture, and color, but they also often define the dish itself. Imagine spaghetti and meatballs without spaghetti sauce or pizza without pizza sauce!

As for salad dressings, there are many excellent bottled versions. However, some compensate for their low-fat content by adding extra sugar, making them more like syrup than dressing. Also, many contain chemicals, preservatives, and other ingredients that might be unsafe for people on a gluten-free diet.

But the best part is you can enjoy all of these tastes and flavors, knowing that the sauces and dressings presented here are wheat-free and gluten-free. They're so delicious that your family and friends will never know!

Apricot Sauce

This sauce is versatile. You can use it to baste Cornish game hens as they bake or to drizzle over pork chops. Toss it with fresh fruit or put it on French toast; just omit the thyme and salt if you use the sauce on fruit.

MAKES ¾ CUP; 4 SERVINGS

½ cup apricot preserves
¼ cup water
½ teaspoon dried thyme
2 tablespoons fresh orange juice
½ teaspoon salt

Heat all the ingredients in a small saucepan over medium heat, stirring constantly, until preserves melt and mixture is blended. Cool before using.

Per serving
CALORIES: 125 FAT: 0.5g PROTEIN: <1g CARBOHYDRATES: 29g
SODIUM: 16mg CHOLESTEROL: 0mg FIBER: 0.5g

■ ■ ■

Avocado Chile Sauce

Avocados may not be part of your everyday repertoire, but this sauce is great with the Southwestern Crab Cakes (page 137). Thinned down a bit with water, it becomes a delicious salad dressing.

MAKES ABOUT 1½ CUPS; 4 SERVINGS

1 avocado, mashed
1 teaspoon chipotle pepper sauce
1 tablespoon fresh lime juice
¼ cup plain yogurt or 3 tablespoons milk
   (cow, rice, or soy)
2 teaspoons cider vinegar
½ teaspoon salt
1 teaspoon ground cumin, toasted until
   aromatic
1 tablespoon olive oil
½ cup chopped fresh cilantro
¼ cup chopped fresh parsley

Combine all ingredients, except the cilantro and parsley, in a blender or food processor. Pulse on and off until the mixture is not quite smooth. Add the cilantro and parsley and pulse just until combined. Serve the sauce at room temperature.

Per serving
CALORIES: 105 FAT: 9g PROTEIN: 2g CARBOHYDRATES: 5g
SODIUM: 285mg CHOLESTEROL: 0mg FIBER: 2g

■ ■ ■

Enchilada Sauce

Use this tasty sauce in your next enchilada recipe. It will taste so much fresher than the bottled or canned variety.

MAKES 2½ CUPS; 4 SERVINGS

1 tablespoon canola oil

1 small onion, finely chopped

1 small garlic clove, minced

1 (16-ounce) can tomatoes, cut into small pieces, undrained

1 (6-ounce) can tomato paste

1 teaspoon chile powder

½ teaspoon dried oregano

2 tablespoons chopped fresh cilantro

½ teaspoon salt

1 teaspoon sugar or honey

Heat the oil in a medium, heavy saucepan over medium heat. Add the onion and garlic and sauté for 3 to 5 minutes, until the onion is transparent. Add the tomatoes with their juice and the remaining ingredients and bring to a boil. Reduce the heat, cover, and simmer for 5 minutes.

Per serving
CALORIES: 105 FAT: 4g PROTEIN: 3g CARBOHYDRATES: 16g
SODIUM: 624mg CHOLESTEROL: 0mg FIBER: 4g

■ ■ ■

Honey-Mustard Sauce

This sauce is great on fish, especially thick fillets and steaks, such as halibut or yellow-fin tuna. It's also great on grilled chicken.

MAKES ABOUT ½ CUP; 4 SERVINGS

¼ cup Dijonnaise mustard

2 tablespoons honey

¼ cup white grape juice

¼ teaspoon dried thyme

3 tablespoons low-sodium, wheat-free tamari soy sauce

½ teaspoon ground ginger

¼ teaspoon white pepper

Combine all the ingredients in a small, heavy saucepan and cook, uncovered, over low heat, stirring occasionally, for about 5 minutes. Serve warm.

Per serving
CALORIES: 60 FAT: 0.5g PROTEIN: 1g CARBOHYDRATES: 13g
SODIUM: 551mg CHOLESTEROL: 0mg FIBER: 0.5g

■ ■ ■

Hollandaise Sauce

I love eggs Benedict, but the traditional Hollandaise sauce is loaded with fat and calories. I've developed this alternate version with a lower fat and calorie content. I think you'll agree; this is a winner!

MAKES 1 CUP; 4 SERVINGS

2 large egg yolks
1 cup nonfat cream cheese, softened, or soft silken tofu
2 tablespoons fresh lemon juice
1/2 teaspoon xanthan gum
2 tablespoons butter or margarine (see note, page 23)
1/4 teaspoon salt
1/8 teaspoon cayenne pepper
1/8 teaspoon white pepper
1/4 teaspoon dry mustard (see note, page 68)

1. Blend the egg yolks, cream cheese, lemon juice, and xanthan gum in a blender until light and fluffy. Transfer the egg yolk mixture to the top of a double boiler set over simmering, not boiling, water. (Don't let the bottom of the double boiler touch the water.) Add the butter and cook, whisking constantly, until the butter has melted and the mixture thickens.

2. Remove from the heat and stir in the remaining ingredients. (The mixture can be kept warm over simmering water for about 30 minutes. If it starts to separate, add 1 teaspoon boiling water and whisk briskly until smooth.)

Per serving
CALORIES: 150 FAT: 8g PROTEIN: 12g CARBOHYDRATES: 5g
SODIUM: 555mg CHOLESTEROL: 130mg FIBER: 0g

■ ■ ■

Tandoori Sauce

*W*hen this marinade is used on meat or chicken it gives a somewhat reddish look after cooking. If you prefer to work with ground spices, use 1/2 teaspoon dried spices for each teaspoon of the cumin, coriander, and mustard seeds.

MAKES ABOUT 1 1/3 CUPS, ENOUGH TO
MARINATE 2 POUNDS OF MEAT; 6 SERVINGS

2 teaspoons cumin seeds
1 teaspoon coriander seeds
1 teaspoon mustard seeds
1 tablespoon sweet paprika
1/2 teaspoon cayenne pepper
1/2 teaspoon ground turmeric
1/2 teaspoon salt
1/2 cup plain yogurt (cow or soy)
2 tablespoons fresh lime juice
1 small onion, chopped
4 garlic cloves, minced
1 tablespoon peeled, grated fresh ginger

1. In a dry heavy skillet, toast the cumin, coriander, and mustard seeds over medium heat, shaking the skillet frequently, for about 5 minutes, or until fragrant. Transfer the spices to a clean coffee grinder (or use a mortar and pestle) and grind the spices to a powder. Add the paprika, cayenne, turmeric, and salt; stir until blended.

2. In a blender or food processor, combine the yogurt, lime juice, onion, garlic, and ginger; purée until smooth. Add the spices and pulse to combine. Use immediately to marinate chicken, meat, or fish.

_____

Per serving
CALORIES: 30 FAT: 0.5g PROTEIN: 2g CARBOHYDRATES: 5g
SODIUM: 285mg CHOLESTEROL: 0mg FIBER: 0.5g

■ ■ ■

Red Chile Sauce

This sauce is practically a staple in Southwestern cooking. Be sure to use the New Mexico red chile powder, not chile powder, which is actually a mix of different spices.

MAKES 6 SERVINGS

3 tablespoons New Mexico red chile powder
  (see note below)
¼ teaspoon salt
1 teaspoon ground white pepper
½ teaspoon ground cumin
½ teaspoon dried oregano
½ teaspoon ground coriander
Dash ground cinnamon
Dash ground cloves
3 cups low-sodium, gluten-free chicken broth
¼ teaspoon Lea & Perrins Worcestershire
  sauce
1 garlic clove, minced
1 tablespoon canola oil
2 tablespoons sweet rice flour or
  white rice flour

1. In a dry heavy saucepan, heat the chile powder, salt, pepper, cumin, oregano, coriander, cinnamon, and cloves over medium heat, stirring constantly, 3 to 5 minutes, or until the spices darken slightly and are fragrant. This lightly toasts the spices, bringing out their flavor.

2. Stir in 2¾ cups of the broth, the Worcestershire sauce, garlic, and oil. Simmer, covered, for 5 to 10 minutes.

3. In a small bowl or cup, combine the rice flour and the remaining ¼ cup broth; stir to form a paste. Add the paste to the sauce and cook, stirring constantly, until the mixture comes to a boil and thickens slightly.

_____

Per serving
CALORIES: 65 FAT: 4g PROTEIN: 6g CARBOHYDRATES: 6g
SODIUM: 397mg CHOLESTEROL: 0mg FIBER: 2g

Note: I use the Dixon brand medium-hot chile powder. You may want to start with only 1 tablespoon of this chile powder or choose a milder chile powder. If you like a hotter sauce, you can always add more to taste.

▪ ▪ ▪

Red Wine Sauce

Serve this sauce over beef or pork. It provides sophisticated, complex flavors.

MAKES ABOUT ¾ CUP; 4 SERVINGS

1 teaspoon canola oil

1 onion, finely chopped

1 garlic clove, minced

1½ cups dry red wine

½ teaspoon Dijonnaise mustard

¼ teaspoon sugar

¼ teaspoon dried thyme

¼ teaspoon dried rosemary

¼ teaspoon dried marjoram

¼ teaspoon ground black pepper

¼ teaspoon salt

1. Heat the oil in a medium, heavy saucepan over medium heat. Add the onion and garlic and sauté for 5 minutes.

2. Add the remaining ingredients; increase the heat to medium-high and cook, uncovered, for about 15 minutes, until the liquid reduces by half.

Per serving
CALORIES: 75 FAT: 0.5g PROTEIN: 1g CARBOHYDRATES: 4g
SODIUM: 283mg CHOLESTEROL: 0mg FIBER: 0.5g

VARIATION

Nonalcoholic Sauce
Substitute pure white grape juice for the red wine. Add 2 tablespoons red wine vinegar and 1 teaspoon fresh lemon juice. Omit the sugar.

▪ ▪ ▪

Lemon-Tomato Barbecue Sauce

I've been making this sauce for nearly thirty years. It's gone through many renditions, but it's basically a very light sauce that is especially good on grilled chicken. My guests always rave about it.

MAKES ABOUT 1 CUP; 6 SERVINGS

1 (6-ounce) can tomato juice

1 small garlic clove, minced

½ teaspoon onion powder

1 teaspoon grated lemon zest

½ teaspoon ground black pepper

1 teaspoon Lea & Perrins Worcestershire sauce

¼ cup fresh lemon juice

1 tablespoon butter or canola oil

Dash cayenne pepper

1. Combine all the ingredients in a small, heavy saucepan and bring to a boil over medium heat. Reduce the heat to low and simmer, uncovered, for 5 minutes.

2. Baste chicken with the sauce during the last 10 minutes of cooking on the grill.

Per serving

CALORIES: 25 FAT: 2g PROTEIN: 1g CARBOHYDRATES: 3g SODIUM: 137mg CHOLESTEROL: 5mg FIBER: 0.5g

■ ■ ■

Green Chile Sauce

*F*or many of us living in the Southwest, this is a sauce we eat often to get our chile "fix." If you're using fresh green chiles, remember that green chiles vary in hotness. Start out with half a chile and sample the sauce. Add more to taste.

MAKES ABOUT 2 CUPS; 4 SERVINGS

1 teaspoon canola oil

$\frac{1}{2}$ cup finely diced onion

1 garlic clove, minced

2 cups low-sodium, gluten-free chicken broth

2 medium green chiles or $\frac{1}{2}$ (4-ounce) can, drained

2 large plum tomatoes, diced

$\frac{1}{2}$ teaspoon ground coriander

$\frac{1}{2}$ teaspoon ground oregano

2 tablespoons chopped fresh cilantro

$\frac{1}{4}$ teaspoon salt

2 teaspoons cornstarch mixed with
   1 tablespoon water

1. Heat the oil in a heavy skillet over medium heat. Add the onion and sauté for 3 to 5 minutes, until tender. Add all the remaining ingredients, except the cornstarch mixture, and simmer, covered, for 15 to 20 minutes.

2. Stir the cornstarch mixture. Add to the sauce and bring to a boil, stirring constantly. Boil, stirring, until the mixture thickens slightly.

Per serving

CALORIES: 70 FAT: 4g PROTEIN: 7g CARBOHYDRATES: 8g SODIUM: 475mg CHOLESTEROL: 0mg FIBER: 1g

■ ■ ■

Barbecue Sauce

*M*y guests have marveled over this rich, thick, barbecue sauce for nearly twenty years now, and it remains a Fenster family favorite. I use it on baby back pork ribs, but it also works on beef.

MAKES 2 CUPS; 8 SERVINGS

1 cup ketchup

$\frac{1}{2}$ cup molasses

2 tablespoons instant chopped onion

2 tablespoons light brown sugar

1 tablespoon mustard seeds

1 teaspoon crushed red pepper

1 teaspoon dried oregano

½ teaspoon black pepper

2 teaspoons sweet paprika

1 teaspoon chile powder

½ teaspoon salt

1 bay leaf

1 garlic clove, minced

1 teaspoon grated orange zest

½ cup fresh orange juice

¼ cup olive oil

¼ cup red wine vinegar

2 tablespoons Lea & Perrins Worcestershire sauce

Combine all the ingredients in a small saucepan and bring to a boil over medium heat. Reduce the heat and simmer, uncovered, for 20 minutes. Discard the bay leaf.

Per serving

CALORIES: 180 FAT: 8g PROTEIN: 1g CARBOHYDRATES: 29g SODIUM: 54mg CHOLESTEROL: 0mg FIBER: 1g

■ ■ ■

Spaghetti Sauce

I've been making this sauce for years, and even though we've tried several others it remains our family favorite. A slow cooker works best; however, you can simmer it on the stovetop if you wish. Just watch it carefully so it doesn't scorch; you may have to add more water to thin it down a bit.

MAKES 12 SERVINGS

1 (48-ounce) can tomato juice

3 (6-ounce) cans tomato paste

3 tablespoons dried parsley

2 tablespoons dried basil

1 tablespoon dried rosemary

2 bay leaves

2 teaspoons dried oregano

½ teaspoon ground black pepper

3 tablespoons sugar

2 teaspoons salt, or to taste

¼ cup grated Romano cheese (optional)

Combine all the ingredients in a large slow cooker; mix well. Cook on medium-low heat, stirring occasionally, all day.

Per serving

CALORIES: 85 FAT: 1g PROTEIN: 4g CARBOHYDRATES: 17g SODIUM: 825mg CHOLESTEROL: 2mg FIBER: 3g

■ ■ ■

Pizza Sauce

This no-fat sauce boasts loads of flavor and is perfect with my Pizza crust (page 147).

MAKES ABOUT 1 CUP, ENOUGH FOR A 12-INCH PIZZA; 6 SERVINGS

1 (8-ounce) can tomato sauce
½ teaspoon dried oregano
½ teaspoon dried basil
½ teaspoon dried rosemary
½ teaspoon fennel seeds
¼ teaspoon garlic powder or 1 garlic
   clove, minced
2 teaspoons sugar
½ teaspoon salt

Combine all the ingredients in a small saucepan and bring to a boil over medium heat. Reduce the heat to low and simmer, uncovered, for 15 minutes. Use the sauce to top a pizza crust.

___

Per 2 to 3 tablespoons
CALORIES: 28 FAT: 0g PROTEIN: 1g CARBOHYDRATES: 7g
SODIUM: 610mg CHOLESTEROL: 0mg FIBER: 1g

■ ■ ■

Tomatillo-Apple Salsa

Tomatillos look like green tomatoes with papery husks. They are found in the produce section. Combined with fresh apples, they are the basis for a great, slightly unusual salsa for grilled chicken or fish.

MAKES 4 SERVINGS

5 tomatillos, husked, rinsed, and chopped
1 yellow bell pepper, chopped
1 small Red Delicious apple, unpeeled, cored
   and chopped
½ cup chopped red onion
¼ cup chopped fresh cilantro
1 tablespoon fresh lemon juice
1 small jalapeño chile, seeded and minced
¼ teaspoon ground cumin
½ teaspoon salt
¼ teaspoon ground white pepper

Mix all the ingredients together in a medium bowl, cover, and refrigerate for up to 3 hours. Serve at room temperature.

___

Per serving
CALORIES: 63 FAT: 1g PROTEIN: 2g CARBOHYDRATES: 14g
SODIUM: 272 mg CHOLESTEROL: 0mg FIBER: 2g

■ ■ ■

Tomatillo Sauce

This is a typical Southwestern sauce that you can use in the same way you'd use a red or green chile sauce: on burritos, eggs, and so on.

MAKES ABOUT 1 CUP; 4 SERVINGS

1 pound tomatillos, husked and rinsed

1 teaspoon olive oil

1 cup chopped onion

1 cup low-sodium, gluten-free chicken broth

1 garlic clove, minced

1 serrano chile, minced

4 teaspoons cider vinegar

1/4 teaspoon dried oregano

1/4 teaspoon ground cumin

1/4 teaspoon sugar or honey

1/2 cup chopped fresh cilantro

1. Preheat the oven to 350°F. Grease a pie plate. Place the tomatillos in the prepared pie plate and bake for 30 minutes, or until the tomatillos are soft but not split. Set aside to cool, then cut into quarters.

2. Meanwhile, heat the oil in a heavy skillet over medium heat. Add the onion and sauté until golden brown. Add the tomatillos, broth, garlic, chile, vinegar, oregano, cumin, and sugar; bring to a boil. Reduce the heat, cover, and simmer for 15 minutes. Cool slightly.

3. Transfer the mixture to a blender. Add all but 2 teaspoons of the cilantro and purée until smooth. Stir in the remaining cilantro.

Per 1/4 cup
CALORIES: 55 FAT: 0.5g PROTEIN: 1g CARBOHYDRATES: 12g
SODIUM: 270mg CHOLESTEROL: 0mg FIBER: 2g

■ ■ ■

White Dill Sauce with Mushrooms

This is a perfect topping for thick-fleshed fish such as halibut or yellow-fin tuna. It's also great on chicken dishes, such as chicken Kiev.

MAKES ABOUT 3/4 CUP; 4 SERVINGS

1 teaspoon canola oil

1/2 cup finely chopped onion

2 cups fresh mushrooms, sliced

1/3 cup low-sodium, gluten-free chicken broth

1 cup milk (cow, rice, or soy)

1/4 teaspoon sugar

1/2 teaspoon dry mustard (see note, page 68)

1/2 teaspoon salt

1/4 teaspoon ground white pepper

2 teaspoons dried dill weed

1 tablespoon cornstarch mixed with

1 tablespoon water

1. Heat the oil in a heavy nonstick saucepan over medium heat. Add the onion and mushrooms and sauté for about 5 minutes. Add the remaining ingredients, except the dill and cornstarch mixture. Bring the mixture to a boil over high heat, stirring constantly. Reduce the heat to medium and cook, uncovered, until the mixture is reduced by half, about 15 minutes. Stir in the dill.

2. Stir the cornstarch mixture until well blended and smooth. Stir the mixture into the sauce and cook, stirring constantly, until the sauce thickens slightly. The sauce is best if served immediately.

Per 3 tablespoons
CALORIES: 70 FAT: 3g PROTEIN: 4g CARBOHYDRATES: 8g
SODIUM: 416mg CHOLESTEROL: 8mg FIBER: 0.5g

■ ■ ■

Cream Sauce for Vegetables

Creamed vegetables remind me of home-style cooking. My mother and mother-in-law always served fresh spring vegetables like sweet green peas in a cream sauce, but it also works on fresh asparagus or carrots.

MAKES ABOUT 1 CUP; 4 SERVINGS

1 cup milk (cow, rice, or soy)
1 tablespoon butter or canola oil
$\frac{1}{4}$ teaspoon salt

$\frac{1}{8}$ teaspoon ground white pepper
2 tablespoons sweet rice flour

1. Heat $\frac{3}{4}$ cup of the milk, the butter, salt, and pepper in a medium saucepan over medium heat.

2. Stir the flour into the remaining $\frac{1}{4}$ cup milk until well blended and smooth. Gradually whisk the flour mixture into the milk mixture and cook, whisking, until the mixture thickens.

Per serving
CALORIES: 80 FAT: 5g PROTEIN: 24g CARBOHYDRATES: 6g
SODIUM: 163mg CHOLESTEROL: 8mg FIBER: 0g

■ ■ ■

Papaya Chutney

This is an unusual yet very tasty version of chutney. Try it with roast chicken, grilled fish, or pork.

MAKES ABOUT 1½ CUPS; 4 SERVINGS

1 teaspoon olive oil
$\frac{1}{2}$ cup diced red onion
1 tablespoon peeled grated fresh ginger
1 small garlic clove, minced
1 teaspoon ground cumin
$\frac{1}{2}$ teaspoon crushed red pepper
$\frac{1}{2}$ cup fresh lime juice
$\frac{1}{4}$ cup packed light brown sugar

1 cup diced papaya

²⁄₃ cup diced plum tomatoes

¹⁄₄ teaspoon salt

¹⁄₈ teaspoon ground white pepper

1 cup chopped fresh cilantro

1. Heat the oil in a heavy skillet over medium-low heat. Add the onion and sauté until slightly tender. Add the ginger, garlic, cumin, and crushed red pepper and cook for 2 minutes. Add the lime juice and brown sugar and simmer until the sauce is thick enough to coat the back of a spoon.

2. Add the papaya and tomatoes and cook just until tender. Add the salt, pepper, and cilantro. Serve at room temperature.

Per serving

CALORIES: 80 FAT: 2g PROTEIN: 1g CARBOHYDRATES: 17g SODIUM: 120mg CHOLESTEROL: 0mg FIBER: 1g

■ ■ ■

Pineapple Salsa

*H*mmm—pineapple on fish? At first, I was a bit dubious about this one, but it's delicious. Try it and you'll agree.

MAKES 2 CUPS; 6 SERVINGS

2 cups chopped fresh or canned pineapple in juice

2 tablespoons finely chopped red onion

2 tablespoons rice vinegar

1 tablespoon sugar or honey

1 small jalapeño chile, stem end removed and seeded

Dash salt

¹⁄₂ cup chopped fresh cilantro

1. Combine all the ingredients, except the cilantro, in a heavy saucepan over medium heat and bring to a boil. Reduce the heat and simmer gently for 10 minutes, or until the mixture thickens slightly. Remove from the heat.

2. Discard the jalapeño chile. Stir in the cilantro. Serve on grilled fish.

Per ¹⁄₃ cup

CALORIES: 25 FAT: 0.5g PROTEIN: 1g CARBOHYDRATES: 7g SODIUM: 1mg CHOLESTEROL: 0mg FIBER: 0.5g

■ ■ ■

Teriyaki Sauce

I know it's hard to find a gluten-free teriyaki sauce, so keep this easy version on hand, and you'll always be prepared. I like to use it for marinating steak, chicken, and shrimp or in any recipe that requires teriyaki sauce.

MAKES 1¹⁄₄ CUPS; 6 SERVINGS

1 cup low-sodium, wheat-free tamari soy sauce

¹⁄₄ cup fresh lemon juice

¼ cup packed light brown sugar

1 teaspoon ground ginger

¼ teaspoon onion powder

¼ teaspoon garlic powder

Combine all the ingredients in a screw-top jar and shake vigorously to blend. Use the sauce to marinate chicken, beef, or pork for at least 4 hours or overnight in the refrigerator. Cook as directed in your recipe. The sauce can be stored in an airtight container in the refrigerator for up to 5 days.

Per ¼ cup

CALORIES: 50 FAT: .5g PROTEIN: 2g CARBOHYDRATES: 9g SODIUM: 1,290mg CHOLESTEROL: 0mg FIBER: 0.5g

▪ ▪ ▪

Apple Chutney

This chutney goes especially well with pork tenderloin (page 153). Even though it has a lot of ingredients, it's well worth the effort. My guests rave about it, and your house will smell heavenly from the aroma!

MAKES 3½ CUPS; 14 SERVINGS

3 cups chopped, peeled Granny Smith apples (about 4)

1 cup chopped onion

¾ cup packed light brown sugar

½ cup cider vinegar

1 cup water

¼ cup finely chopped red bell pepper

¼ cup finely chopped yellow bell pepper

½ cup golden raisins

1 tablespoon peeled grated fresh ginger

1 garlic clove, minced

¼ teaspoon crushed red pepper

1¼ teaspoons salt

½ teaspoon ground ginger

¼ teaspoon ground nutmeg

¼ teaspoon ground allspice

⅛ teaspoon ground cloves

⅛ teaspoon ground white pepper

1. In a large, heavy saucepan, combine the apples, onion, sugar, vinegar, water, bell peppers, raisins, grated ginger, garlic, crushed red pepper, 1 teaspoon of the salt, ground ginger, nutmeg, allspice, and cloves. Bring to a boil over medium heat, stirring until the sugar has dissolved.

2. Reduce the heat and simmer, uncovered, for 1 hour. Add the remaining ¼ teaspoon salt and white pepper. Remove from the heat and set aside to cool. Store in the refrigerator for up to 1 week. Serve warm or at room temperature.

Per ¼ cup

CALORIES: 65 FAT: 0.5g PROTEIN: 1g CARBOHYDRATES: 17g SODIUM: 16mg CHOLESTEROL: 0mg FIBER: 1g

▪ ▪ ▪

Yogurt Cheese

This is one of the best innovations in low-fat cooking! It is so simple, yet it produces the smooth, creamy texture we all crave, without all the fat or calories. This method can be used with flavored yogurts as well, but yogurts with gelatin will not drain as thoroughly (if at all). I prefer to use a brand that has a high acidophilus content.

MAKES ¾ CUP; 4 SERVINGS

1 (8-ounce) carton low-fat plain yogurt

1. Place a coffee filter inside a strainer and place the strainer over a bowl or measuring cup. Spoon the yogurt into the coffee filter. Place a plastic bag around the strainer and bowl so that it's sealed from the air. Refrigerate for 3 hours or overnight. (The longer the yogurt drains the firmer it becomes.)

2. Discard the liquids that collect in the bottom of the bowl. Store the cheese in the refrigerator for about 5 days.

Per 3 tablespoons
CALORIES: 32 FAT: 0.5g PROTEIN: 3g CARBOHYDRATES: 4g
SODIUM: 43mg CHOLESTEROL: 1mg FIBER: 0g

■ ■ ■

Asian Vinaigrette

A great dressing to serve over rice vermicelli or a combination of butter lettuce and mandarin oranges.

MAKES ABOUT ⅔ CUP; 6 SERVINGS

1 tablespoon low-sodium, wheat-free
tamari soy sauce
2 tablespoons Teriyaki Sauce (page 92)
4 teaspoons fresh lime juice
1 tablespoon honey
2 tablespoons olive oil
2 tablespoons sesame oil
2 tablespoons Lea & Perrins Worcestershire
sauce

In a screw-top jar, combine all the ingredients. Cover and shake vigorously until blended. Refrigerate, covered, for up to 1 week.

Per 2 tablespoons
CALORIES: 60 FAT: 5g PROTEIN: 1g CARBOHYDRATES: 5g
SODIUM: 210mg CHOLESTEROL: 0mg FIBER: 0.5g

■ ■ ■

Avocado Dressing

This is a very tasty dressing for plain old lettuce, and it complements a Southwestern meal quite nicely.

MAKES 1 CUP; 8 SERVINGS

1 large ripe avocado
$\frac{1}{4}$ cup water
1 teaspoon fresh lime juice
$\frac{1}{8}$ teaspoon grated lime zest
$\frac{1}{2}$ teaspoon grated fresh onion
$\frac{1}{8}$ teaspoon ground cumin
1 small garlic clove, minced
$\frac{1}{8}$ teaspoon ground white pepper

Peel, pit, and mash the avocado in a small bowl. Combine the avocado and the remaining ingredients in a food processor or blender. Process until desired consistency. This dressing is best if served immediately.

Per 2 tablespoons
CALORIES: 30 FAT: 3g PROTEIN: 1g CARBOHYDRATES: 2g
SODIUM: 3mg CHOLESTEROL: 0mg FIBER: 1g

■ ■ ■

Buttermilk Dressing

This is great on any lettuce salad, but it's especially good on the first tender leaf lettuce from your garden.

MAKES ABOUT 1$\frac{1}{2}$ CUPS; 12 SERVINGS

$\frac{1}{4}$ teaspoon ground black pepper
$\frac{1}{2}$ teaspoon onion salt
1 teaspoon dried chives
$\frac{1}{8}$ teaspoon xanthan gum
1 cup buttermilk or 2 tablespoons cider vinegar
   and enough milk (cow, rice, or soy) to equal
   1 cup
2 tablespoons red wine vinegar
2 teaspoons Dijonnaise mustard
1 small garlic clove, minced

Stir the pepper, onion salt, chives, and xanthan gum in a screw-top jar until blended. Add the remaining ingredients, cover tightly, and shake vigorously to blend. Refrigerate, covered, for up to 1 week.

Per 2 tablespoons
CALORIES: 10 FAT: .5g PROTEIN: 1g CARBOHYDRATES: 1g
SODIUM: 100mg CHOLESTEROL: 1mg FIBER: 0.5g

■ ■ ■

Citrus Dressing

Fennel and basil add a refreshing note to this citrus-flavored dressing, which goes especially well with fish or chicken entrées.

MAKES ½ CUP; 4 SERVINGS

2 teaspoons fennel seeds, toasted
¼ teaspoon crushed red pepper
⅛ teaspoon salt
⅛ teaspoon xanthan gum
Dash ground white pepper
2 tablespoons rice vinegar
2 tablespoons olive oil
2 tablespoons finely chopped fresh basil
¼ cup fresh orange juice
1 tablespoon grated orange zest
2 teaspoons fresh lime juice
2 teaspoons grated lime zest

Combine the fennel seeds, crushed red pepper, salt, xanthan gum, and pepper in a screw-top jar. Shake vigorously to mix. Add the remaining ingredients, cover tightly, and shake to blend thoroughly. Refrigerate, covered, for up to 1 week.

Per 2 tablespoons
CALORIES: 50 FAT: 5g PROTEIN: 1g CARBOHYDRATES: 2g
SODIUM: 45mg CHOLESTEROL: 0mg FIBER: 0.5g

Hazelnut Vinaigrette

Delicate oils like hazelnut are a taste treat and are great in salad dressings such as this one. Buy flavored oils in small quantities, store them in a dark place, and use them up quickly.

MAKES ABOUT 1 CUP; 8 SERVINGS

1 tablespoon fresh snipped chives or 1 teaspoon dried chives
1 teaspoon sugar
¼ teaspoon ground black pepper
⅛ teaspoon xanthan gum
¼ cup hazelnut oil
¼ cup water
¼ cup white wine vinegar
2 tablespoons fresh lemon juice
1 tablespoon Dijonnaise mustard

Combine the chives, sugar, pepper, and xanthan gum in a screw-top jar. Cover and shake well. Add the remaining ingredients, cover tightly, and shake well to blend. Refrigerate, covered, for up to 2 weeks.

Per 2 tablespoons
CALORIES: 65 FAT: 7g PROTEIN: 1g CARBOHYDRATES: 2g
SODIUM: 24mg CHOLESTEROL: 0mg FIBER: 0.5g

Herb Vinaigrette

The nice thing about making your own vinaigrettes is that you can control what goes into them. This one also doubles as a marinade for fish or chicken before it goes on the grill.

MAKES ABOUT 1 CUP; 8 SERVINGS

$\frac{1}{2}$ teaspoon dry mustard (see note, page 68)
1 tablespoon dried parsley
$\frac{1}{2}$ teaspoon dried chives
$\frac{1}{4}$ teaspoon dried chervil
$\frac{1}{4}$ teaspoon powdered sugar
$\frac{1}{8}$ teaspoon xanthan gum
$\frac{1}{4}$ cup olive oil
$\frac{1}{4}$ cup water
$\frac{1}{4}$ cup red wine vinegar

Combine the mustard, herbs, sugar, and xanthan gum in a screw-top jar. Cover and shake vigorously. Add the oil, water, and vinegar, cover tightly, and shake until well blended. Refrigerate, covered, for up to 1 week.

Per 2 tablespoons
CALORIES: 65 FAT: 7g PROTEIN: 1g CARBOHYDRATES: 1g
SODIUM: 1 mg CHOLESTEROL: 0mg FIBER: 0.5g

■ ■ ■

Lime-Cilantro Dressing

Lime and cilantro are two of my favorite flavors. This is a perfect dressing for a salad accompanying a Southwestern meal.

MAKES ABOUT 1 CUP; 8 SERVINGS

$\frac{1}{2}$ teaspoon salt
$\frac{1}{2}$ teaspoon powdered sugar
$\frac{1}{8}$ teaspoon ground cumin
$\frac{1}{8}$ teaspoon xanthan gum
1 teaspoon grated lime peel
$\frac{1}{4}$ cup fresh lime juice
$\frac{1}{4}$ cup chopped fresh cilantro
$\frac{1}{2}$ cup olive oil
$\frac{1}{4}$ cup water
$\frac{1}{4}$ cup rice vinegar
1 small garlic clove, minced

Combine the salt, sugar, cumin, and xanthan gum in a screw-top jar. Add the remaining ingredients, cover, and shake vigorously until well blended. Refrigerate, covered, for up to 1 week.

Per 2 tablespoons
CALORIES: 65 FAT: 7g PROTEIN: 1g CARBOHYDRATES: 2g
SODIUM: 135mg CHOLESTEROL: 0mg FIBER: 0.5g

■ ■ ■

Peanut Dressing

This is the perfect dressing for pure buckwheat noodles or Thai-style pasta.

MAKES ½ CUP; 4 SERVINGS

2 tablespoons olive oil
1 tablespoon gluten-free peanut butter
   (commercial, not freshly ground)
1 tablespoon low-sodium, wheat-free tamari
   soy sauce
3 tablespoons rice vinegar
1 tablespoon water
1 teaspoon light brown sugar
⅛ teaspoon crushed red pepper

In a medium bowl, combine all the ingredients. Heat on High power in a microwave for 1 minute, or until the mixture is hot. Stir the mixture until the peanut butter has melted. Serve warm or at room temperature.

――――――――

Per 2 tablespoons
CALORIES: 60 FAT: 5g PROTEIN: 1g CARBOHYDRATES: 3g
SODIUM: 140mg CHOLESTEROL: 0mg FIBER: 0.5g

■ ■ ■

Pine Nut Dressing

This is a unique way to use pine nuts, which are almost a staple in the Southwest. I like to leave some of the pine nuts in chopped form to add some texture.

MAKES ½ CUP; 4 SERVINGS

¼ cup pine nuts, toasted (see page 52)
¼ cup red or pink grapefruit juice
2 teaspoons white wine vinegar
2 tablespoons fresh orange juice
¼ teaspoon powdered sugar
⅛ teaspoon salt
⅛ teaspoon xanthan gum
Dash ground white pepper
2 tablespoons olive oil

In a blender, combine all the ingredients, except the oil, and blend until smooth. With the motor running, slowly add the oil in a thin stream and continue blending until the dressing has thickened. Refrigerate, covered, for up to 1 week.

――――――――

Per 2 tablespoons
CALORIES: 110 FAT: 11g PROTEIN: 2g CARBOHYDRATES: 4g SODIUM: 67mg CHOLESTEROL: 0mg FIBER: 0.5g

■ ■ ■

Raspberry Vinaigrette

Salad dressings with raspberry vinegar are very popular these days. When you taste this one, you'll see why. It's great!

MAKES 1¼ CUPS; 10 SERVINGS

¼ cup fresh raspberries

¼ cup raspberry vinegar (see note, below)

¼ cup pure white grape or apple juice

¼ cup fresh lemon juice

¼ cup water

1 teaspoon Dijonnaise mustard

1 teaspoon sugar

½ teaspoon onion powder

¼ teaspoon salt

⅛ teaspoon xanthan gum

¼ cup olive oil

Press the raspberries through a sieve into a bowl; discard the seeds. Combine all the ingredients, except the oil, in a blender. With the motor running, slowly add the oil in a thin stream and continue blending until the dressing has thickened. Refrigerate, covered, for up to 2 days.

Per 2 tablespoons
CALORIES: 60 FAT: 5g PROTEIN: 1g CARBOHYDRATES: 2g
SODIUM: 60mg CHOLESTEROL: 0mg FIBER: 0.5g

Note: If you can't find raspberry vinegar, make your own: Place 2 raspberry-flavored herbal tea bags in ¼ cup rice vinegar or cider vinegar. Let steep at room temperature for 2 to 3 hours.

■ ■ ■

Red Chile Dressing

Be sure to use red chile powder, preferably from New Mexico, not chile powder, which is actually a mix of several spices.

MAKES ABOUT 1 CUP; 8 SERVINGS

¼ cup water

1 tablespoon cider vinegar

1 tablespoon fresh lemon juice

1 tablespoon Lea & Perrins Worcestershire sauce

2 teaspoons Dijonnaise mustard

1 garlic clove, minced

1 teaspoon red chile powder

½ teaspoon Reese anchovy paste

½ teaspoon sweet paprika

⅛ teaspoon xanthan gum

¼ cup olive oil

Combine all the ingredients, except the oil, in a food processor or blender. With the motor running, slowly add the oil in a thin stream and continue blending until the dressing has thickened. Refrigerate, covered, for up to 1 week.

Per 2 tablespoons

CALORIES: 65 FAT: 7g PROTEIN: 1g CARBOHYDRATES: 1g SODIUM: 48mg CHOLESTEROL: 0mg FIBER: 0.5g

■ ■ ■

Southwestern Dressing

A very simple yet flavorful way to dress salad greens in Southwestern style.

MAKES ABOUT ¼ CUP; 4 SERVINGS

1 teaspoon chile powder

1 teaspoon dried oregano

1 teaspoon ground cumin, toasted until aromatic

¼ teaspoon ground black pepper

⅛ teaspoon xanthan gum

¼ cup red wine vinegar

2 tablespoons olive oil

Combine the chile powder, oregano, cumin, pepper, and xanthan gum in a screw-top jar. Add the vinegar and oil, cover tightly, and shake vigorously to blend well.

Per 1 tablespoon

CALORIES: 65 FAT: 7g PROTEIN: 1g CARBOHYDRATES: 2g SODIUM: 7mg CHOLESTEROL: 0mg FIBER: 0.5g

■ ■ ■

Thousand Island Dressing

This dressing is a critical component of Reuben sandwiches, some of my favorites. It's the preferred dressing for those who like creamy salad dressings.

MAKES 2 CUPS; 16 SERVINGS

1 cup low-fat mayonnaise

3 tablespoons cocktail sauce

1 tablespoon finely chopped green bell pepper

1 tablespoon finely chopped red bell pepper

1 teaspoon dried chives

Blend all the ingredients in a bowl with a wire whisk. Refrigerate, covered, for up to 1 week.

Per 2 tablespoons

CALORIES: 200 FAT: 22g PROTEIN: 1g CARBOHYDRATES: 1g SODIUM: 157mg CHOLESTEROL: 16mg FIBER: 0g

■ ■ ■

Walnut Oil Vinaigrette

Walnut oil makes a special vinaigrette to dress salad greens, especially when combined with oranges. It also tastes great on cooked Brussels sprouts, making a vegetable that isn't necessarily everyone's favorite a new taste experience.

MAKES ABOUT ½ CUP; 4 SERVINGS

½ teaspoon dried thyme leaves
¼ teaspoon salt
⅛ teaspoon ground black pepper
⅛ teaspoon xanthan gum
½ cup walnut oil
¼ fresh orange juice
2 teaspoons balsamic vinegar

Combine the thyme, salt, pepper, and xanthan gum in a screw-top jar, cover, and shake to blend. Add the oil, juice, and vinegar. Cover tightly and shake vigorously until well blended. Refrigerate, covered, for up to 1 week.

Per 2 tablespoons
CALORIES: 130 FAT: 14g PROTEIN: 1g CARBOHYDRATES: 2g SODIUM: 134mg CHOLESTEROL: 0mg FIBER: 0.5g

■ ■ ■

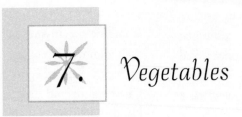

7. Vegetables

e all know we should include more vegetables in our diets because they are good sources of important nutrients and fiber. Unfortunately, gluten-sensitive people do not always know the components of the sauces, thickeners, or seasonings often found on the prepared vegetables in restaurants, in other people's homes, or in prepackaged vegetables at the grocery store.

You'll notice that there aren't many recipes in this section. That's because there are many ways to eat vegetables without using flour. You can eat them raw, of course, or cooked and topped with Parmesan cheese or herbs, or glazed with a little sugar, maple syrup, or flavored oil, but this excludes some of our favorite vegetable dishes.

This chapter concentrates on recipes that would typically include wheat, either as a binder or thickener. Family favorites such as Scalloped Potatoes, Hash-Brown Casserole, and Creamed Corn are featured.

Creamed Corn

Creamed corn is an all-American food, the perfect accompaniment for a meal of roast chicken or roast beef.

MAKES 4 SERVINGS

1 teaspoon cornstarch
1 cup water
$\frac{1}{2}$ teaspoon salt
2 teaspoons sugar
$\frac{1}{8}$ teaspoon ground white pepper
1 cup fresh or frozen corn kernels

1. Combine the cornstarch with 2 tablespoons of the water in a small bowl and stir until well blended. Add the remaining water and the cornstarch mixture to a medium saucepan. Cook, stirring constantly, over medium heat until the mixture has thickened. Remove from the heat. Add the salt, sugar, and pepper.

2. Add the corn. Purée some of the corn either with a handheld immersion blender or in a blender. If using a handheld blender, blend the contents of the saucepan until about half of the corn is puréed, leaving some whole kernels. If using a blender, add half of the corn mixture to the blender and pulse on and off to the desired consistency. Return the mixture to the saucepan. Heat to serving temperature.

Per serving
CALORIES: 45 FAT: 0.5g PROTEIN: 1g CARBOHYDRATES: 11g
SODIUM: 270mg CHOLESTEROL: 0mg FIBER: 1g

■ ■ ■

Eggplant Parmesan

Imagine my dismay to learn that the eggplant Parmesan I thought was safe in restaurants actually contains wheat bread crumbs. Some of you may enjoy my version as a meatless main dish, but it's also great just as a vegetable side dish.

MAKES 4 SERVINGS

3 tablespoons balsamic vinegar
1 tablespoon olive oil
$\frac{1}{2}$ teaspoon salt
$\frac{1}{2}$ teaspoon sugar or honey
$\frac{1}{4}$ teaspoon dried oregano
$\frac{1}{4}$ teaspoon dried basil
$\frac{1}{2}$ teaspoon ground black pepper
1 $\frac{1}{2}$ pounds eggplant, unpeeled, cut crosswise
    into $\frac{1}{2}$-inch-thick slices
2 $\frac{1}{2}$ cups Spaghetti Sauce (page 88)
4 ounces mozzarella cheese or nondairy
    cheese, shredded
1 tablespoon greated Parmesan cheese (cow or
    soy), plus additional for garnish (optional)
Fresh basil leaves (optional)

1. Preheat the oven to 400°F. Grease a baking sheet. Combine the vinegar, oil, salt, sugar, oregano, basil, and pepper in a bowl. Dip each eggplant slice into the mixture and arrange in single layer on the prepared baking sheet. Bake for 15 minutes per side, or until tender. Leave the oven on.

2. Grease a shallow 2-quart baking dish. Spoon ¾ cup of the sauce into the prepared dish. Arrange half of the eggplant over the sauce. Spoon ¾ cup of the sauce over the eggplant. Sprinkle with half of the mozzarella cheese. Arrange the remaining eggplant over the sauce. Top with the remaining sauce and end with the remaining mozzarella and Parmesan cheese.

3. Cover with foil and bake for 20 minutes. Uncover and bake for another 15 minutes, or until bubbly. Let stand for 15 minutes before serving for easier cutting. Garnish with additional Parmesan cheese and basil leaves, if desired.

Per serving

CALORIES: 220 FAT: 10g PROTEIN: 8g CARBOHYDRATES: 25g SODIUM: 811mg CHOLESTEROL: 11mg FIBER: 6g

■ ■ ■

Hash-Brown Casserole

This dish falls into the comfort food category. It tastes good, the texture is pleasing, and it reminds me of old-fashioned, home-cooked meals. This recipe is dairy-based.

MAKES 6 SERVINGS

¾ cup chopped onion

1½ tablespoons tapioca flour

¼ teaspoon dry mustard (see note, page 68)

¼ teaspoon salt

¼ teaspoon ground white pepper

¼ cup low-sodium, gluten-free chicken broth

½ cup skim milk (cow, rice, or soy)

½ cup shredded sharp Cheddar cheese

¼ cup shredded Swiss cheese

½ cup Yogurt Cheese (page 94) or ⅓ cup
   plain yogurt

1 pound purchased gluten-free hash-brown
   potatoes, thawed, or grated fresh potatoes

Sweet paprika, for garnish

1. Preheat the oven to 350°F. Grease an 8-inch-square pan.

2. Coat a medium saucepan with cooking spray. Add the onion and cook, covered, over medium-low heat for 3 minutes, or until tender. Combine the flour, mustard, salt, pepper, broth, and milk in a screw-top jar and shake until well blended (or blend in a blender). Add to the onion and cook, stirring, 5 min-

utes, or until the mixture thickens. Remove from the heat. Add the Cheddar and Swiss cheeses and stir until the cheeses have melted. Stir in the Yogurt Cheese.

3. Combine the cheese mixture and potatoes. Spread in prepared pan. Sprinkle with paprika. Cover and bake for 30 minutes; uncover and bake for 20 minutes longer. Serve immediately.

_____

Per serving

CALORIES: 225 FAT: 11g PROTEIN: 8g CARBOHYDRATES: 22g SODIUM: 628mg CHOLESTEROL: 14mg FIBER: 0.5g

■ ■ ■

Hot German Potato Salad

I'm a big fan of German food, and this is a great side dish for smoked pork chops or roast pork. The combination of sweet and tart flavors is very tantalizing.

MAKES 4 SERVINGS

2 pounds new potatoes

1 strip lean bacon

$\frac{1}{2}$ cup light brown sugar

$\frac{1}{2}$ cup cider vinegar

1 teaspoon Dijonnaise mustard

$\frac{3}{4}$ teaspoon celery seeds

1 tablespoon grated onion

$\frac{1}{2}$ teaspoon salt

$\frac{1}{4}$ teaspoon ground black pepper

$\frac{1}{4}$ cup chopped green bell pepper

$\frac{1}{4}$ cup diced red bell pepper

1 tablespoon chopped fresh parsley, for garnish

1. Peel the potatoes and cook in boiling water to cover for about 15 minutes, or until tender. Cool slightly and cut into $\frac{3}{4}$-inch cubes. Transfer the potatoes to a large serving dish.

2. Meanwhile, fry the bacon in a skillet over medium heat until crisp. With a slotted spoon, transfer the bacon to paper towels to drain.

3. Add the sugar, vinegar, mustard, celery seeds, onion, salt, black pepper, and bell peppers to the bacon drippings. Cook, stirring, over medium heat until the mixture comes to a boil. Reduce the heat and simmer for 1 minute.

4. Crumble the bacon and stir into the sauce. Pour the sauce over the potatoes and toss with a spatula until well coated. Sprinkle with the parsley. Serve warm.

_____

Per serving

CALORIES: 160 FAT: 1g PROTEIN: 2g CARBOHYDRATES: 40g SODIUM: 61mg CHOLESTEROL: 1mg FIBER: 1g

■ ■ ■

Oven-Fried Potatoes

These potatoes are crispy on the outside and soft on the inside. Best of all they're super simple. Rosemary is a natural complement to potatoes, but I also like to use the same amount of thyme or savory leaves for a change.

MAKES 4 SERVINGS

2 large baking potatoes, cut lengthwise into
    8 wedges
½ tablespoon olive oil
½ teaspoon sweet paprika
½ teaspoon dried rosemary leaves, crushed
½ teaspoon salt

1. Preheat the oven to 400°F. Grease a baking sheet. Place the potato wedges in a plastic bag or bowl. Add the oil. Toss or shake until evenly coated with oil. Add the paprika, rosemary, and salt. Shake or toss to coat.

2. Arrange the potatoes on the prepared baking sheet in a single layer. Bake for 30 minutes, or until the potatoes are nicely browned on all sides, turning frequently for even browning.

――――――――――

Per serving
CALORIES: 60 FAT: 2g PROTEIN: 1g CARBOHYDRATES: 10g
SODIUM: 6mg CHOLESTEROL: 0mg FIBER: 1g

Potato Pancakes

In some circles, these tasty little pancakes are called potato latkes. They're great topped with applesauce or sour cream.

MAKES 4 SERVINGS

2 cups grated, peeled potatoes
    (4 medium potatoes)
1 large egg, well beaten
2 tablespoons white rice flour
1 teaspoon baking powder
1 teaspoon salt
¼ teaspoon ground white pepper
½ small onion, grated
1 tablespoon olive oil

1. Combine all the ingredients, except the oil, in a large bowl.

2. Heat a skillet or griddle over medium heat until hot. Add the oil. Using ¼ cup for each pancake, drop the batter onto the hot griddle. Cook for 5 to 7 minutes on each side, until golden brown.

――――――――――

Per serving
CALORIES: 90 FAT: 5g PROTEIN: 3g CARBOHYDRATES: 12g
SODIUM: 710mg CHOLESTEROL: 53mg FIBER: 0.5g

Note: Assemble all other ingredients before grating the potatoes. Work quickly once the potatoes are grated to prevent them from discoloring.

■ ■ ■

Scalloped Potatoes

This is another of those comfort-food dishes, the kind we occasionally crave. Bake it in the same oven while the Best-Ever Meat Loaf (page 145) cooks or add ham for a meal in itself.

MAKES 4 SERVINGS

4 medium russet potatoes, peeled and sliced

¾ teaspoon onion salt

¼ teaspoon ground white pepper

1 tablespoon instant chopped onion

⅛ teaspoon ground nutmeg

½ teaspoon dry mustard (see note, page 68)

1 tablespoon canola oil

2 tablespoons potato starch or sweet rice flour

2 cups skim or 1% milk (or rice or soy milk)

1 tablespoon grated Parmesan cheese
   (cow or soy; optional)

1 tablespoon butter or margarine
   (see note, page 23), diced

Sweet paprika, for garnish

1. Preheat the oven to 350°F. Grease a 1½-quart casserole or baking dish. Toss the potatoes with the onion salt, pepper, and onion in the casserole.

2. Combine the remaining ingredients, except the butter and paprika, in a screw-top jar. Shake vigorously until the ingredients are thoroughly blended or blend in a blender until smooth. Pour the milk mixture over the potatoes. Dot with the butter. Lightly sprinkle with paprika. Bake uncovered for 1 hour, or until the sauce is bubbly and the potatoes are lightly browned.

Per serving

CALORIES: 185 FAT: 7g PROTEIN: 7g CARBOHYDRATES: 25g SODIUM: 400mg CHOLESTEROL: 10mg FIBER: 2g

VARIATION

Scalloped Potatoes with Ham

Add 1 cup cubed ham in step 1 and reduce the onion salt to ½ teaspoon.

■ ■ ■

Grilled Vegetables and Quinoa

One of the greatest flavor combinations is fresh vegetables and the smoky, charcoal flavor from the grill. If grilling is not possible, stir-fry the vegetables in a skillet.

MAKES 6 SERVINGS

MARINADE

2 tablespoons olive oil

1/3 cup balsamic vinegar

1/3 cup chopped green onions

1/2 teaspoon dried oregano leaves

1 garlic clove, minced

1/2 teaspoon ground coriander

1/4 teaspoon ground cumin

1/4 teaspoon salt

1/4 teaspoon ground black pepper

2 teaspoons molasses

VEGETABLES

4 carrots, peeled and halved lengthwise

1 large red bell pepper

1 large yellow bell pepper

4 red new potatoes, halved

2 medium zucchini, cut crosswise into 1/4-inch-thick rounds

1 large onion, halved

2 small yellow squash, cut crosswise into 1/4-inch-thick rounds

2 cups cooked quinoa or brown rice

1. To make the marinade: Combine all the ingredients in a large bowl. Set aside.

2. To prepare the vegetables: Cut the vegetables into large pieces, keeping the thickness to about 1/4 inch, thin enough to cook thoroughly yet thick enough to remain whole during the process. Add the vegetables to the marinade, stir to coat, and let stand for 30 to 45 minutes, stirring occasionally.

3. Drain the vegetables and arrange in a grill basket that has been coated with cooking spray. Reserve the marinade.

4. Grill the vegetables over medium-hot coals with the lid closed for 15 to 20 minutes, turning every 5 minutes. Meanwhile, bring the marinade to a boil over medium heat.

5. Remove the vegetables from the grill basket; transfer to a bowl and toss with the hot marinade. Serve warm with quinoa.

Per serving
CALORIES: 140 FAT: 5g PROTEIN: 4g CARBOHYDRATES: 24g SODIUM: 207mg CHOLESTEROL: 0mg FIBER: 4g

■ ■ ■

8. *Main Dishes*
Poultry

Poultry, especially chicken, is one of the most versatile foods in our diets. It can take on a variety of different personalities, depending on how it's prepared—grilled, roasted, or baked—and the sauces we put on it can very from hot and spicy to mellow and creamy.

In this section, chicken is prepared in a variety of ways for the gluten-sensitive person. Skinless, boneless chicken breasts are featured in many of these dishes. They are extremely low in fat and very easy to prepare because there is no skin or bones to remove. You can substitute other chicken pieces in most of these recipes, however, the fat and calorie content will increase.

In this chapter, I also offer a few ideas for breading and binding foods together. While breading isn't used only with chicken, I offer them here because it seems that many chicken dishes require dredging in flour or in a seasoned breading mix or binding. With my suggestions, you'll know what flours to use and what to do.

Breading and Binding Ideas for Fried Meats, Fish, Poultry, and Vegetables

If there's one question that usually perplexes new gluten-free cooks, it's "What can I use in place of wheat flour for breading, dredging, and binding?" We're all used to reaching for the wheat flour to coat foods before frying, and bread crumbs are our first choice for binding dishes such as meat loaf, crab cakes, or croquettes. I've listed some of my favorite breading and binding ideas below.

Fried meats, fish, and vegetables can be breaded with any of the following. Dip in milk, buttermilk, or beaten egg first. Each breading produces a different texture and taste, so experiment a little to see what you like.

Amaranth flakes (www.NuWorldAmaranth.com)
Cornflakes (Nature's Path)
Cornmeal (Quaker)
Cream of rice cereal (Gerber)
Crushed corn tortilla chips
Crushed or finely ground nuts, such as almonds
Crushed nut crackers (Blue Diamond)
Crushed rice crackers (Edward and Sons)
Gluten-free bread crumbs
Mashed potato flakes
Quinoa flakes
Southern Homestyle cornflake crumbs*
Southern Homestyle tortilla crumbs*

To dredge food in a single flour (or in a combination of unseasoned flours) before frying, I prefer using flours made of sorghum, quinoa, corn (not cornstarch), and amaranth. Quinoa and amaranth have stronger flavors that might affect the flavor of your dish, so you might want to mix them with a more neutral flour such as sorghum. They also tend to brown more quickly, so mixing them with sorghum flour reduces that tendency as well.

---

*New from Bethel Grain Company, Benton, IL; ask your grocer to order them.

Flours such as arrowroot and tapioca do not make good single-flour dredging choices, because they tend to get sticky and gummy. Cornstarch is best when used with other flours (such as cornmeal), but it can be used alone for a very light coating. For more information on individual flours, see pages 229–42.

Versatile Breading Mix

With the basic proportions below, you can use this breading mix on many different foods. I like the combination of thyme, savory, and oregano for poultry. For an Italian twist, use the basil, oregano, and rosemary. Fish responds nicely to dill and parsley. Vary the herbs to your liking. If you're wondering why there is sugar in the mix, it balances the flavors and promotes browning.

MAKES 2 CUPS; 32 TABLESPOONS

1 cup yellow or white cornmeal

1 cup cornstarch or sorghum flour

1 teaspoon dried thyme or basil

1 teaspoon dried parsley, oregano, or dill weed

1 teaspoon dried savory or dried crushed
   rosemary

1 teaspoon onion powder

1 teaspoon sweet paprika

1 teaspoon salt or seasoned salt

$1/2$ teaspoon cayenne pepper

$1/4$ teaspoon garlic powder

$1/4$ teaspoon sugar

Mix all the ingredients together. Use as breading mix for meats, seafood, or vegetables in frying and baking. Do not reuse mix after dipping raw meat into it. Store in an airtight container in a dark, dry place; use within 3 months.

Per tablespoon
CALORIES: 35 FAT: 0g PROTEIN: 1g CARBOHYDRATES: 8g
SODIUM: 80mg CHOLESTEROL: 0mg FIBER: 1g

■ ■ ■

Chicken and Broccoli Quiche

Looking more like a custard than a quiche, this dish eliminates the traditional pastry crust. Fat content is further reduced by using ricotta cheese and yogurt, with a minimal amount of Swiss cheese. This recipe is dairy based.

MAKES 6 SERVINGS

1 cup low-fat ricotta cheese

$1/2$ cup plain low-fat yogurt

2 medium eggs

¼ cup brown rice flour

½ teaspoon baking powder

⅛ teaspoon ground nutmeg

½ teaspoon celery salt

¼ cup grated Parmesan cheese (cow or soy)

1½ cups chopped cooked chicken

1 (10-ounce) package frozen broccoli, thawed and drained

¼ cup shredded Swiss cheese

1. Preheat the oven to 350°F. Grease a 9-inch pie plate.

2. Combine the ricotta cheese, yogurt, eggs, flour, baking powder, nutmeg, celery salt, and Parmesan cheese in a blender and purée until smooth. Transfer to a large bowl. Stir in the chicken and broccoli. Spoon into the prepared pie plate and top with the Swiss cheese.

3. Bake for 30 to 45 minutes, or until a toothpick inserted near the center comes out clean. Let stand for 10 minutes before serving.

Per serving

CALORIES: 250 FAT: 12g PROTEIN: 22g CARBOHYDRATES: 11g SODIUM: 349mg CHOLESTEROL: 131mg FIBER: 2g

■ ■ ■

Chicken Breasts with Mushrooms

I've been making this recipe for over twenty years, having converted it from one given to me by my dear friend Pat Grantier. Thanks, Pat. If you use a nondairy cheese, it may not melt as nicely as regular cheese.

MAKES 4 SERVINGS

4 boneless, skinless chicken breast halves

¾ cup dried gluten-free bread crumbs

½ teaspoon dried thyme

2 tablespoons brown rice flour

3 large eggs, lightly beaten

½ teaspoon salt

¼ teaspoon ground black pepper

2 tablespoons olive oil

1 cup sliced fresh mushrooms

½ cup shredded provolone or Muenster cheese or nondairy cheese of your choice

½ cup dry white wine

⅓ cup fresh lemon juice

1. Rinse the chicken and pat dry with paper towels. Cut into thin slices.

2. Combine the bread crumbs (a good way to use up your leftover gluten-free bread), thyme, and flour in a pie plate. Dip the chicken pieces into the eggs, then the crumb mixture. Season with salt and pepper.

3. Preheat the oven to 350°F. Grease an 8-inch-square baking dish.

4. Heat the oil in a heavy skillet over medium heat. Add the chicken and sauté on both sides until golden brown.

5. Arrange the chicken in a single layer in the prepared baking dish, top with the mushrooms, and sprinkle the cheese on top. Pour in the wine. Bake for 30 to 40 minutes or until the cheese melts and the liquid bubbles. Before serving, drizzle the lemon juice over the casserole.

Per serving
CALORIES: 350 FAT: 13g PROTEIN: 30g CARBOHYDRATES: 21g SODIUM: 35mg CHOLESTEROL: 61mg FIBER: 1g

■ ■ ■

Chicken Tandoori

The tangy flavors of this dish remind one of faraway, exotic places. And, its brilliant red-orange color looks gorgeous on your plate.

MAKES 4 SERVINGS

1 tablespoon olive oil

1 medium onion, diced

1 garlic clove, minced

2 teaspoons ground coriander

2 teaspoons ground cumin

2 teaspoons ground turmeric

2 teaspoons sweet paprika

1 tablespoon grated fresh ginger

1 tablespoon red wine vinegar

1 teaspoon salt

¼ teaspoon cayenne pepper

1 (8-ounce) carton plain yogurt or ½ to ⅔ cup nondairy milk (rice or soy)

2 teaspoons grated lemon zest

4 chicken legs (drumsticks and thighs)

1 small lemon, sliced

¼ cup chopped fresh parsley

1. Heat the oil in a small, heavy skillet over medium heat. Add the onion and sauté for 1 minute. Add the garlic, coriander, cumin, turmeric, paprika, ginger, vinegar, salt, and cayenne. Cook, stirring frequently, for about 10 minutes, or until the onion is tender and well coated with spices. Remove from the heat; cool for 5 minutes.

2. In a large bowl, combine the onion mixture, yogurt, and lemon zest. Rinse the chicken and pat dry with paper towels. Add to the yogurt mixture and marinate in the refrigerator for up to 4 hours.

3. Preheat the oven to 425°F. Grease a shallow baking dish. Remove the chicken from the marinade, reserving the marinade, and arrange the chicken in a single layer in the prepared baking pan. Bake, uncovered, for 45 minutes, turning once. Brush with reserved marinade during the last 5 minutes of baking. Garnish with the lemon and parsley.

Per serving
CALORIES: 430 FAT: 15g PROTEIN: 60g CARBOHYDRATES:
12g SODIUM: 967mg CHOLESTEROL: 228mg FIBER: 1g

▪ ▪ ▪

Chicken Shepherd's Pie

This dish is a great way to use up leftover chicken (or turkey), mashed potatoes, and vegetables. I often make it a couple of days after a holiday meal to use up those final leftovers lurking in my refrigerator.

MAKES 4 SERVINGS

1 cup green peas

1 cup chopped carrots

¼ cup corn kernels

1 tablespoon canola oil

1 small onion, chopped

2 celery stalks, chopped

1 garlic clove, minced

2½ cups low-sodium, gluten-free chicken broth

2 tablespoons tapioca flour mixed with
　3 tablespoons water

1 pound cooked chicken or turkey, cubed

½ cup sliced fresh mushrooms

½ teaspoon celery salt

½ cup dry white wine

1 teaspoon dried thyme

⅓ cup chopped fresh parsley

2 cups mashed potatoes

2 tablespoons grated Parmesan cheese
(cow or soy)

1. Preheat the oven to 450°F. Cook the peas, carrots, and corn in a small amount of boiling, salted water until crisp-tender. Set aside.

2. Heat the oil in a medium skillet over medium heat. Add the onion, celery, and garlic and sauté until the onion is transparent. Add the broth and bring to a boil. Reduce the heat and simmer for about 5 minutes, or until the mixture is reduced by one-third.

3. Stir the tapioca flour mixture and slowly stir into the onion mixture. Simmer, stirring constantly, until the mixture has thickened. Add the reserved vegetables and all the remaining ingredients, except the potatoes and Parmesan cheese.

4. Spoon the mixture into 4 individual soup bowls. Mound the mashed potatoes on top, covering the surface entirely. Sprinkle with the Parmesan cheese. Bake for about 35 minutes, or until the potatoes are browned.

Per serving
CALORIES: 420 FAT: 10g PROTEIN: 41g CARBOHYDRATES:
37g SODIUM: 1,750mg CHOLESTEROL: 72mg FIBER: 4g

▪ ▪ ▪

Turkey Mole

There are many different versions of mole (pronounced MOH-lay). This one has the unmistakable flavor of the Southwest. Yes, that's chocolate you see in the ingredients. It adds a level of complexity that's characteristic of mole, yet you won't be able to distinguish it from all the other flavors.

MAKES 6 SERVINGS

1 cup slivered almonds

1 cup chopped onion

1 small garlic clove, minced

½ teaspoon ground cinnamon

½ teaspoon ground cloves

½ teaspoon ground coriander

¼ teaspoon crushed red pepper

⅛ teaspoon fennel seeds, crushed

1 cup low-sodium, gluten-free chicken broth

2 medium tomatoes, chopped

½ cup chopped fresh cilantro

¼ teaspoon ground black pepper

1 (4-ounce) can diced green chiles, drained

¼ cup raisins

1 ounce unsweetened chocolate, melted

1 (2-pound) cooked turkey breast

1. In a blender, combine all the ingredients except the chocolate and turkey; purée until smooth. Add the chocolate and blend until combined.

2. Place the turkey in a Dutch oven or large skillet. Pour the sauce over the turkey breast. Cover and simmer over low heat for 20 minutes, or until the turkey is heated through.

3. To serve, cut the turkey diagonally into slices. Transfer the slices to dinner plates and top with the sauce.

_____

Per serving

CALORIES: 310 FAT: 19g PROTEIN: 23g CARBOHYDRATES: 19g SODIUM: 165mg CHOLESTEROL: 34mg FIBER: 4g

VARIATION

Chicken Peanut Mole

Substitute 4 cooked boneless, skinless chicken breasts for the turkey breast. Add 2 tablespoons creamy gluten-free peanut butter or nut butter of choice to the sauce.

_____

Per serving

CALORIES: 320 FAT: 19g PROTEIN: 23g CARBOHYDRATES: 19g SODIUM: 165mg CHOLESTEROL: 34mg FIBER: 4g

■ ■ ■

Chicken Cacciatore

The aroma of this dish wafting through the house on a cold, winter day is intoxicating. A crisp lettuce salad and crusty French Bread (page 25) complete the dinner.

MAKES 4 SERVINGS

1 tablespoon olive oil

4 boneless, skinless chicken breast halves

3 cups fresh mushrooms, trimmed and halved

1 small green bell pepper, chopped

1 large onion, sliced

1 garlic clove, minced

½ cup dry red wine

1 (28-ounce) can chopped tomatoes, undrained

2 tablespoons tomato paste

2 tablespoons fresh lemon juice

2 teaspoons dried basil

1 teaspoon sugar

1 teaspoon dried thyme

¼ teaspoon crushed red pepper

½ teaspoon salt

¼ teaspoon ground black pepper

2 teaspoons cornstarch mixed with
   2 tablespoons water

2 cups cooked purchased gluten-free pasta
   (penne or rotini)

1. Heat the oil in a large, heavy skillet or Dutch oven over medium heat. Add the chicken and brown on all sides. Remove the chicken from the skillet and set aside. Add the mushrooms, bell pepper, onion, and garlic to the skillet. Cook, stirring occasionally, until the vegetables are tender.

2. Add the wine and bring to a boil. Reduce the heat and simmer, uncovered, until the liquid has nearly evaporated. Add the tomatoes with their juice, tomato paste, lemon juice, basil, sugar, thyme, crushed red pepper, salt, and black pepper.

3. Return the chicken to the pan and simmer, uncovered, for 15 minutes. Stir the cornstarch mixture. Add the mixture to the sauce and cook, stirring constantly, until the sauce has thickened.

Per serving

CALORIES: 190 FAT: 4g PROTEIN: 17g CARBOHYDRATES: 18g SODIUM: 470mg CHOLESTEROL: 40mg FIBER: 3g

■ ■ ■

Chicken Curry

The spices and apricots make this dish full of very interesting flavors.

MAKES 4 SERVINGS

1 tablespoon canola oil

1 small onion, chopped

1 garlic clove, minced

4 boneless, skinless chicken breast halves

½ cup water

1½ teaspoons ground coriander

1 teaspoon ground ginger

½ teaspoon ground cardamom

¾ teaspoon ground cumin

¼ teaspoon ground turmeric (optional)

¼ teaspoon cayenne pepper

½ cup golden raisins

¼ cup apricot preserves

2 tablespoons cornstarch mixed with
   2 tablespoons water

½ teaspoon salt

¼ teaspoon ground black pepper

1 cup plain yogurt or ⅔ cup nondairy milk

Sweet paprika, for garnish

Cooked rice (optional)

1. Heat the oil in a large, heavy skillet over medium heat. Add the onion and garlic and sauté until lightly browned. Add the chicken and sauté until browned on both sides. Add the water, spices, raisins, and apricot preserves. Simmer, covered, for 10 to 15 minutes, stirring occasionally.

2. Stir the cornstarch mixture. Add the cornstarch mixture, salt, and pepper to the skillet and stir to combine. Simmer, stirring constantly, until the sauce thickens. Gently stir in the yogurt and heat to serving temperature, but do not boil. Garnish each serving with paprika. Serve alone or over cooked rice, if you like.

Per serving

CALORIES: 295 FAT: 5g PROTEIN: 25g CARBOHYDRATES: 37g SODIUM: 519mg CHOLESTEROL: 52mg FIBER: 2g

■ ■ ■

Creamed Chicken on Biscuits

Save those leftover biscuits and top them with this flavorful sauce. Leftover chicken works great, too! This recipe is dairy based, unless you use one of the sour cream alternatives found in health food stores.

MAKES 4 SERVINGS

1 tablespoon canola oil

4 boneless, skinless chicken breast halves, cut into 1-inch cubes

4 cups fresh mushrooms, trimmed and halved

½ cup chopped onion

1 garlic clove, minced

½ cup low-sodium, gluten-free chicken broth

½ teaspoon celery salt

¼ teaspoon ground white pepper

2 tablespoons cornstarch

1 cup gluten-free sour cream or sour cream alternative

1 cup skim milk (cow, rice, or soy)

8 biscuits (page 206)

4 tablespoons finely chopped green onions or chives, for garnish

1. Heat the oil in a large, heavy skillet over medium heat. Add the chicken and sauté, stirring occasionally, for 5 to 7 minutes, until cooked through. Remove the chicken from the pan and set aside.

2. Add the mushrooms, onion, and garlic. Cook, uncovered, for 5 to 7 minutes, until the liquid evaporates.

3. Add all but 2 tablespoons of the broth, the celery salt, and pepper to the skillet. Stir the cornstarch into the 2 tablespoons broth to form a paste. Add the paste to the chicken mixture and cook, stirring, over medium heat until bubbly and thickened. Continue to cook, stirring, for 1 minute.

4. In a bowl, combine the sour cream and

milk and stir until blended. Gently stir the sour cream mixture into the skillet. Heat to serving temperature, but do not boil. Serve over biscuits. Garnish with the green onions.

Per serving

CALORIES: 760 FAT: 33g PROTEIN: 36g CARBOHYDRATES: 81g SODIUM: 1,614mg CHOLESTEROL: 113mg FIBER: 1g

■ ■ ■

Chicken Paprikás with Pasta

This dish has a rich, bold flavor that fills the house with a wonderful aroma. Use purchased gluten-free pasta, such as penne or fusilli, or noodles from your own homemade pasta (page 49).

MAKES 4 SERVINGS

2 tablespoons canola oil

4 boneless, skinless chicken breast halves

1 large onion, finely chopped

1 garlic clove, minced

2 tablespoons sweet Hungarian paprika

1 (16-ounce) can tomatoes, drained

1/4 teaspoon cayenne pepper

1/2 teaspoon sugar

1 teaspoon dried thyme

1/2 teaspoon salt

1/4 teaspoon ground black pepper

1 cup trimmed and sliced mushrooms

1 cup low-sodium, gluten-free chicken broth

2 teaspoons cornstarch mixed with
 2 tablespoons water

1/2 cup gluten-free sour cream or sour cream alternative

2 cups cooked purchased gluten-free pasta (penne or fusilli)

1 teaspoon dried parsley

1. Heat the oil in a large, heavy Dutch oven over medium heat. Add the chicken and brown on both sides. Remove the chicken from the pan and set aside.

2. Add the onion to the pan and sauté, stirring occasionally, for 5 minutes. Add the garlic and paprika and cook, stirring constantly, for 1 minute. Stir in the tomatoes, cayenne, sugar, thyme, salt, and black pepper.

3. Return the chicken to the pan, add the mushrooms and broth, and bring to a boil. Reduce the heat, cover, and simmer for 20 minutes. (Can be prepared up to this point, then refrigerated for up to 24 hours.)

4. Stir the cornstarch mixture. Add the mixture to the sauce, and cook 3 minutes, stirring, until the sauce thickens. Gently stir in the sour cream. Serve over the hot pasta. Garnish with the parsley.

Per serving

CALORIES: 500 FAT: 12g PROTEIN: 42g CARBOHYDRATES: 56g SODIUM: 840mg CHOLESTEROL: 123mg FIBER: 4g

■ ■ ■

and golden. Serve immediately, topped with the cilantro.

Per serving

CALORIES: 370 FAT: 25g PROTEIN: 28g CARBOHYDRATES: 8g SODIUM: 435mg CHOLESTEROL: 283mg FIBER: 0.5g

VARIATION

Meatless Chile Relleno Casserole
Omit the chicken.

Per serving

CALORIES: 330 FAT: 23g PROTEIN: 23g CARBOHYDRATES: 8g SODIUM: 420mg CHOLESTEROL: 267mg FIBER: 0.5g

■ ■ ■

Coq au Vin

This is an elegant blend of flavors, and the dish cooks slowly on its own, leaving you free to do other things. I like to serve it with crusty French Bread (page 25) and a tossed salad.

MAKES 4 SERVINGS

4 skinless chicken drumsticks
4 skinless chicken thighs
1 bacon slice
1 teaspoon olive oil
1 (10-ounce) package frozen pearl onions, thawed
½ pound fresh small button mushrooms, trimmed

Chile Relleno Casserole with Chicken

This is a family favorite, combining the delicious flavors of chiles, eggs, and cheese. Omit the chicken for a meatless dish. This recipe is dairy based.

MAKES 4 SERVINGS

1 cup shredded Monterey Jack
1 cup shredded Colby cheese
1 cup cubed, cooked chicken
1 (4-ounce) can diced green chiles, drained
4 large eggs, lightly beaten
1 cup gluten-free light sour cream
½ teaspoon dried oregano
¼ teaspoon ground cumin
⅛ teaspoon chile powder
Sweet paprika, for garnish
¼ cup chopped fresh cilantro

1. Preheat the oven to 350°F. Grease an 8-inch-square glass baking dish. Alternately layer the cheeses, chicken, and chiles (in that order) in the prepared dish, ending with the cheeses.

2. Beat the eggs, sour cream, oregano, cumin, and chile powder in a bowl until combined. Pour over the layers in the baking dish. Sprinkle generously with paprika. Bake for 30 to 45 minutes, or until the top is puffy

1 cup low-sodium, gluten-free chicken broth

½ cup dry red wine

1 teaspoon sugar or honey

1 teaspoon dried thyme

1 teaspoon dried rosemary, crushed

1 teaspoon sweet paprika

½ teaspoon celery salt

½ teaspoon ground black pepper

¼ teaspoon salt

1 garlic clove, peeled

1 pound small new potatoes, scrubbed

1 pound baby carrots

½ cup chopped fresh parsley

1. Preheat the oven to 400°F. Rinse the chicken and pat dry. Cook the bacon in a heavy, ovenproof Dutch oven over medium heat until crisp. With a slotted spoon, transfer the bacon to paper towels to drain.

2. Add the oil to the Dutch oven. Add the chicken and brown over medium heat on all sides. Remove the chicken from the pan and set aside.

3. Add the onions to the pan and cook over medium heat for about 5 minutes. Add the mushrooms and sauté for 5 minutes. Slowly pour in the broth and wine. Add the sugar, thyme, rosemary, paprika, celery salt, pepper, salt, and garlic.

4. Return the chicken to the pan and add the potatoes. Crumble the bacon and add. Bake, covered, for 30 minutes. Reduce the heat to 350°F. Add the carrots and bake for 30 minutes. Check the chicken; it should be nearly falling off the bone. Garnish with the parsley.

Per serving
CALORIES: 310 FAT: 9g PROTEIN: 23g CARBOHYDRATES: 33g
SODIUM: 500mg CHOLESTEROL: 65mg FIBER: 3g

■ ■ ■

Enchiladas

Enchiladas are a classic Mexican dish. There are many versions of this Southwestern staple, so try this one and then improvise as you wish. You can fill them with anything from chopped seafood to shredded pork. This recipe is dairy based, but you can use your favorite nondairy cheeses instead.

MAKES 4 SERVINGS

1 teaspoon light olive oil

1 cup chopped onion

1 garlic clove, minced

1 (16-ounce) can chopped tomatoes, undrained

1 (8-ounce) can tomato sauce

1 (4-ounce) can diced green chiles, drained

½ teaspoon dried basil

½ teaspoon dried oregano

½ teaspoon celery salt

½ teaspoon ground cumin

1 teaspoon sugar

½ cup chopped fresh cilantro, plus
    2 tablespoons, for garnish

1 cup shredded Monterey Jack cheese

1 cup shredded Cheddar cheese,

8 gluten-free corn tortillas

4 boneless, skinless chicken breast halves, cooked and cut each in half

1 cup gluten-free light sour cream or sour cream alternative

1. Heat the oil in a heavy, medium saucepan over medium heat. Add the onion and garlic and sauté for about 4 minutes. Add the tomatoes with their juice, the tomato sauce, chiles, basil, oregano, celery salt, cumin, sugar, and ½ cup cilantro; bring to a boil. Reduce the heat, cover, and simmer for 15 minutes. Remove from the heat.

2. Preheat the oven to 350°F. Grease a 13 x 9-inch baking pan. Combine the cheeses in a bowl. Dip each corn tortilla into the tomato sauce to soften. Place a strip of chicken and 2 tablespoons of the cheese on each tortilla. Roll up and place, seam side down, in the prepared pan.

3. Add the sour cream to the remaining tomato sauce; stir until blended. Pour the sauce over the enchiladas. Top with the remaining cheeses. Bake for 35 minutes, or until heated through. Garnish with the remaining 2 tablespoons cilantro.

Per serving

CALORIES: 665 FAT: 28g PROTEIN: 63g CARBOHYDRATES: 41mg SODIUM: 1,345mg CHOLESTEROL: 170mg FIBER: 6g

VARIATIONS

Beef Enchiladas

Brown ½ pound lean ground beef and substitute it for the chicken.

Per serving

CALORIES: 625 FAT: 37g PROTEIN: 34g CARBOHYDRATES: 41g SODIUM: 1,271mg CHOLESTEROL: 115mg FIBER: 6g

Meatless Enchiladas

Omit the chicken and fill each tortilla with 4 tablespoons of the cheeses.

Per serving

CALORIES: 475 FAT: 25g PROTEIN: 24g CARBOHYDRATES: 41g SODIUM: 1,345mg CHOLESTEROL: 170mg FIBER: 6g

■ ■ ■

Cornish Game Hens with Fruit Glaze

The glaze on these game hens is fabulous and causes them to brown beautifully. This makes an excellent dish for dinner guests because it's both visually stunning and exceedingly tasty.

MAKES 4 SERVINGS

2 Cornish game hens, thawed if frozen, halved

½ teaspoon salt

¼ teaspoon ground black pepper

½ cup raspberry jam

¼ teaspoon dried thyme

¼ teaspoon dried tarragon

1 teaspoon olive oil

¼ cup red wine vinegar

1 garlic clove, minced

1. Preheat the oven to 400°F. Spray a roasting pan with cooking spray. Rinse the game hens with cold water and pat dry with paper towels. Season with the salt and pepper. Arrange the game hens, skin side up, in the prepared pan. (If possible, place them on a roasting rack so they won't sit in their drippings.)

2. Combine the remaining ingredients in a small bowl and microwave on High power until the jam has melted. Stir the mixture thoroughly.

3. Bake the hens, covered, for 45 minutes to 1 hour, brushing two or three times with the glaze. The juices should run clear when the hens are pierced with a knife in the thickest part.

Per serving

CALORIES: 785 FAT: 39g PROTEIN: 77g CARBOHYDRATES: 27g SODIUM: 1,169mg CHOLESTEROL: 248mg FIBER: 0.5g

■ ■ ■

Lemon Chicken

Often found in Chinese restaurants, this dish is extremely simple to prepare at home. If you're serving it on a large platter to dinner guests, garnish the platter with bright red tomatoes or thin slices of red pepper for a dramatic effect.

MAKES 4 SERVINGS

4 boneless, skinless chicken breast halves

½ cup plus 2 tablespoons cornstarch

¾ cup water

2 large egg yolks

2 tablespoons canola oil

3 tablespoons light brown sugar

1 tablespoon peeled grated fresh ginger

1 cup low-sodium, gluten-free chicken broth

⅓ cup fresh lemon juice

1 teaspoon grated lemon zest

½ cup finely chopped green onions

1. Rinse the chicken with cold water and pat dry with paper towels.

2. In a medium bowl, combine ½ cup cornstarch, ¼ cup of the water, and the egg yolks; whisk until smooth. Dip each chicken breast into the batter to coat completely.

3. Heat the oil in a large, heavy skillet over medium heat. Add the chicken and brown on all sides. With a slotted spoon, transfer the chicken to paper towels to drain; keep warm.

4. Add the remaining 1 tablespoon cornstarch, brown sugar, and ginger to the skillet. Stir in the remaining ½ cup water and the broth. Cook over medium heat, stirring frequently, until the mixture thickens and comes to a boil. Remove from the heat. Stir in the

lemon juice and zest. Cook for 15 to 20 minutes or until chicken juices run clear.

5. Cut each chicken breast slightly on a diagonal into 4 pieces. Arrange on a dinner plate and top each with sauce. Sprinkle with the green onions.

Per serving

CALORIES: 320 FAT: 11g PROTEIN: 25g CARBOHYDRATES: 28g SODIUM: 463mg CHOLESTEROL: 158mg FIBER: 0.5g

▪ ▪ ▪

Lemon-Tarragon Chicken

*B*oneless, skinless, chicken breasts are a real timesaver in the kitchen. Here, they are teamed with lemon and tarragon in a creamy sauce and served over pasta.

MAKES 4 SERVINGS

1 tablespoon canola oil

4 boneless, skinless chicken breast halves

1 cup fresh mushrooms, trimmed and halved

1 garlic clove, minced

1½ teaspoons dried tarragon

½ teaspoon ground black pepper

1 (14.5-ounce) can low-sodium, gluten-free chicken broth

2 tablespoons cornstarch

2 tablespoons gluten-free light sour cream or sour cream alternative

1 teaspoon grated lemon zest

4 cups cooked purchased gluten-free pasta (noodles or penne)

2 tablespoons chopped fresh parsley, for garnish

1. Heat the oil in a large, heavy skillet over medium-high heat. Add the chicken, mushrooms, garlic, tarragon, and pepper. Cook, uncovered, for 15 minutes, or until the chicken is no longer pink, turning once. With a slotted spoon, transfer the chicken and mushrooms to a platter and set aside.

2. Combine 2 tablespoons of the broth with the cornstarch in a small bowl. Add the cornstarch mixture and remaining broth to the skillet, and cook, stirring, over medium-high heat until thickened and bubbly.

3. Remove about ½ cup of the mixture and stir it into the sour cream. (If you're using a sour cream alternative, you may need to whisk it into the mixture or put it in a blender to fully incorporate it.) Return the sour cream mixture to the skillet along with the chicken and mushrooms. Stir in the lemon zest. Heat to serving temperature, but do not boil. Serve over hot noodles. Garnish with the parsley.

Per serving

CALORIES: 355 FAT: 9g PROTEIN: 31g CARBOHYDRATES: 33g SODIUM: 805mg CHOLESTEROL: 91mg FIBER: 2g

▪ ▪ ▪

Mexican Chicken Casserole

I've served this dish for years. It features all the classic Mexican flavors in a creamy casserole topped with cheese. You may use nondairy versions of the Monterey Jack and Cheddar cheeses, if you wish. Because they don't melt as nicely as dairy cheeses, you may want to stir all of the cheese into the mixture rather than sprinkling some on top. Garnish with a sprinkle of paprika.

MAKES 6 SERVINGS

1 cup low-sodium, gluten-free chicken broth

1 cup canned Mexican-style tomatoes

1 medium onion, finely diced

½ cup gluten-free light sour cream or sour cream alternative

1 (4-ounce) can diced green chiles, drained

½ teaspoon dried oregano

¼ teaspoon ground sage

¼ teaspoon ground cumin

¼ teaspoon chile powder

¼ teaspoon garlic powder

½ teaspoon salt

2 cups cubed, cooked chicken

1 cup shredded Cheddar cheese

1 cup shredded Monterey Jack cheese

2 cups corn tortilla chips

2 tablespoons chopped fresh cilantro, for garnish

1. Preheat the oven to 350°F. Grease a 14 x 10-inch casserole dish. Mix the broth, tomatoes, onion, sour cream, chiles, oregano, sage, cumin, chile powder, garlic powder, and salt together in a bowl to form a sauce. Set aside.

2. Layer half of the chicken, then half of the sauce, cheeses, and tortilla chips in the prepared dish. Repeat the layers, ending with the cheeses. Bake for 35 to 40 minutes, or until the casserole is bubbly. Garnish with the cilantro.

Per serving

CALORIES: 325 FAT: 18g PROTEIN: 28g CARBOHYDRATES: 15g SODIUM: 688mg CHOLESTEROL: 73mg FIBER: 2g

■ ■ ■

Oven-Fried Chicken

*L*ow-fat and easy as can be! There's no need to stand over an oil-splattering skillet to get crispy fried chicken. Let your oven do the work. Try the spicy version below if you like your fried chicken with a little kick.

MAKES 4 SERVINGS

8 skinless chicken thighs

½ cup buttermilk or 1 teaspoon cider vinegar plus enough nondairy milk to make ½ cup

¼ teaspoon cayenne pepper

¼ teaspoon garlic powder

¼ cup brown rice flour

3 tablespoons cornmeal

½ teaspoon salt

¼ teaspoon ground white pepper

¼ teaspoon sweet paprika

1. Preheat the oven to 400°F. Coat a baking sheet with cooking spray. Rinse the chicken with cold water and pat dry with paper towels.

2. In a pie plate, mix the buttermilk, cayenne, and garlic powder. In another pie plate, mix the remaining ingredients, except the chicken. Dip each chicken thigh into the buttermilk mixture, then into the flour mixture. Place on prepared baking sheet. Gently spray with cooking spray. Bake for 45 to 60 minutes, or until the chicken is crispy and juices run clear.

Per serving

CALORIES: 250 FAT: 7g PROTEIN: 31g CARBOHYDRATES: 14g
SODIUM: 427mg CHOLESTEROL: 124mg FIBER: 1g

VARIATION

Spicy Oven-Fried Chicken
To the flour mixture, add 1 teaspoon *each* dried oregano, dried basil, and dried thyme and ¼ teaspoon cayenne pepper.

■ ■ ■

Tarragon-Dijon Chicken

This dish has never failed to please, and even impress, my guests. They inevitably ask, "What's in this?" The tarragon and thyme marry nicely with the pineapple juice to create a delectable sauce.

MAKES 4 SERVINGS

4 boneless, skinless chicken breast halves

⅔ cup pineapple juice

½ cup dry white wine

1 tablespoon Lea & Perrins Worcestershire sauce

1 tablespoon Dijonnaise mustard

½ teaspoon salt

¼ teaspoon ground black pepper

½ teaspoon dried tarragon

¼ teaspoon dried thyme

1 teaspoon cornstarch mixed with 1 tablespoon water

2 tablespoons chopped fresh parsley, for garnish

1. Preheat the oven to 375°F. Grease an 8-inch-square baking pan. Rinse the chicken with cold water and pat dry with paper towels. Arrange the chicken in the prepared pan.

2. In a small bowl, combine the remaining ingredients, except the cornstarch mixture and parsley, and pour over the chicken. Cover

and bake for 45 to 50 minutes. Uncover, turn the chicken, and bake for 10 minutes longer.

3. Transfer the juices from the baking pan to a saucepan, leaving the chicken in the oven to stay warm. (Use turkey baster to remove the juices.) Stir the cornstarch mixture. Add the cornstarch mixture to the pan juices and cook over medium heat, stirring, until the mixture thickens.

4. To serve, pour one-third of the sauce over the chicken. Garnish with the parsley. Serve the remaining sauce on the side.

Per serving
CALORIES: 150 FAT: 2g PROTEIN: 21g CARBOHYDRATES: 7g
SODIUM: 378mg CHOLESTEROL: 51mg FIBER: 0.5g

■ ■ ■

Thai Chicken

*E*thnic dishes provide us with a great variety of flavor combinations. This one features peanut butter, ginger, and cilantro.

MAKES 4 SERVINGS

¾ cup Teriyaki Sauce (page 92)
¼ cup creamy peanut butter (not freshly ground) or soy nut butter
1 tablespoon sugar
1 teaspoon peeled grated fresh ginger
¼ cup water
½ teaspoon crushed red pepper

2 tablespoons chopped fresh cilantro
4 boneless, skinless chicken breast halves

1. Combine all the ingredients, except the chicken, in the top of a double boiler over simmering water. Stir until smooth, then cook for about 20 minutes, or until the mixture thickens. Cool.

2. Preheat the oven to 350°F. Grease an 8-inch-square baking dish.

3. Rinse the chicken with cold water and pat dry with paper towels. Arrange the chicken in a single layer in the prepared dish; brush the sauce generously over the chicken. Bake for 25 to 30 minutes, or until the chicken is cooked through, basting once with the sauce. Bring any remaining sauce to a boil in a microwave-safe bowl and serve with the chicken.

Per serving
CALORIES: 270 FAT: 10g PROTEIN: 28g CARBOHYDRATES: 18g
SODIUM: 2,899mg CHOLESTEROL: 51mg FIBER: 1g

■ ■ ■

Grilled Chicken with Spicy Glaze

*T*his dish is delicious and very easy. Make the sauce the night before, light the grill when you get home from work the next day, and prepare the remainder of the meal while the chicken cooks.

MAKES 4 SERVINGS

8 pieces skinless chicken legs and thighs

½ teaspoon salt

¼ teaspoon ground black pepper

2 tablespoons Dijonnaise mustard

2 tablespoons molasses

2 tablespoons fresh orange juice

1 tablespoon low-sodium, wheat-free tamari
  soy sauce

1 tablespoon grated fresh ginger

1 teaspoon grated orange zest

1. Preheat a grill. Rinse the chicken with cold water and pat dry with paper towels. Season the chicken with the salt and pepper. Grill the chicken, turning as needed.

2. While the chicken is grilling, mix the remaining ingredients together in a small bowl. When the chicken starts to brown, baste with the glaze and grill, basting occasionally for about 20 minutes, or until the chicken is cooked through.

Per serving
CALORIES: 210 FAT: 5g PROTEIN: 29g CARBOHYDRATES: 8g
SODIUM: 607mg CHOLESTEROL: 113mg FIBER: 0.5g

■ ■ ■

Grilled Chicken with Ancho Chile Sauce

Ancho chiles are dried poblano chiles; they provide a mild, yet definite "heat" to the sauce. If anchos are unavailable locally, try Mail-Order Sources (page 257).

MAKES 4 SERVINGS

4 boneless, skinless chicken breast halves

1½ teaspoons salt

¼ teaspoon ground black pepper

1½ cups water

1 dried ancho chile

1 garlic clove, peeled

½ teaspoon dried thyme

½ cup fresh orange juice

1 tablespoon sugar

1 teaspoon olive oil

1. Rinse the chicken with cold water and pat dry with paper towels. Season the chicken with ½ teaspoon of the salt and the pepper. Preheat a grill or broiler. Grill the chicken, turning as needed, for about 20 minutes, or until cooked through.

2. While the chicken is cooking (or up to 1 day before serving), combine the water, chile, garlic, remaining 1 teaspoon salt, and thyme in a saucepan over medium heat and bring to a boil; boil for about 5 minutes.

3. Using a slotted spoon, remove the chile and garlic from the cooking liquid. Reserve the cooking liquid. Discard the stem from the chile and remove the seeds. Purée the chile and garlic in a blender or food processor. With the motor running, add ½ cup of the cooking liquid, the orange juice, sugar, and oil and purée until the mixture is smooth. Serve the sauce with chicken.

Per serving

CALORIES: 140 FAT: 3g PROTEIN: 20g CARBOHYDRATES: 7g SODIUM: 863mg CHOLESTEROL: 51mg FIBER: 0.5g

■ ■ ■

Grilled Chicken with Peach Salsa

Fresh peaches combined with fragrant spices top this grilled chicken. This dish is especially nice in summer, when peaches are in season. It's a great way to get extra fruit into your diet.

MAKES 4 SERVINGS

4 boneless, skinless chicken breast halves

½ teaspoon salt

¼ teaspoon ground black pepper

4 medium ripe peaches

1 tablespoon fresh lemon juice

¼ teaspoon celery salt

1 cup chopped red bell pepper

1 small onion, chopped

¼ teaspoon cayenne pepper

1 teaspoon ground cumin

⅓ cup packed light brown sugar

⅓ cup cider vinegar

2 tablespoons diced green chiles

⅓ cup chopped fresh cilantro

1. Rinse the chicken with cold water and pat dry with paper towels. Season the chicken with the salt and pepper. Preheat a grill or broiler. Grill the chicken, turning as needed, for about 20 minutes, or until cooked through.

2. While the chicken is cooking, peel, pit, and cut the peaches into thin wedges. Toss with the lemon juice and celery salt. Set aside.

3. In a heavy skillet coated with cooking spray, sauté the bell pepper and onion, stirring occasionally, for about 5 minutes, or until the vegetables are crisp-tender. Add the cayenne and cumin and stir for 1 minute. Add the sugar and vinegar and cook, stirring occasionally, for about 3 minutes. Add the peach mixture (including juices) and chiles and heat until hot. Stir in the cilantro. Serve at room temperature over the chicken.

Per serving

CALORIES: 210 FAT: 2g PROTEIN: 22g CARBOHYDRATES: 27g SODIUM: 572mg CHOLESTEROL: 51mg FIBER: 3g

■ ■ ■

❋Grilled Chicken with Teriyaki Glaze

This dish is easy and very tasty—great for summertime grilling. The fennel lends an interesting note.

MAKES 4 SERVINGS

4 boneless, skinless chicken breast halves
½ teaspoon salt
¼ teaspoon ground black pepper
½ cup Teriyaki Sauce (page 92)
2 teaspoons balsamic vinegar
½ teaspoon fennel seed, toasted
½ teaspoon grated orange zest

1. Rinse the chicken with cold water and pat dry with paper towels. Season the chicken with the salt and pepper. Preheat a grill or broiler.

2. Combine the remaining ingredients in a small bowl. Grill the chicken, turning as needed and brushing frequently with the sauce for about 20 minutes, or until cooked through.

Per serving
CALORIES: 130 FAT: 2g PROTEIN: 22g CARBOHYDRATES: 6g SODIUM: 1,707mg CHOLESTEROL: 51mg FIBER: 0.5g

❋Grilled Chipotle Chicken

Chipotles are dried, smoked jalapeño chiles and are *very* hot, but they make great sauces when used in the right amount. If they're not available in your area, check the Mail-Order Sources (page 257).

MAKES 4 SERVINGS

4 boneless, skinless chicken breast halves
1 dried whole chipotle, soaked in ¼ cup boiling water for 30 minutes
¼ cup fresh orange juice
1 teaspoon Dijonnaise mustard
1 tablespoon cider vinegar
1 tablespoon molasses
¼ teaspoon salt

1. Preheat a grill. Rinse the chicken with cold water and pat dry with paper towels.

2. Discard the chile and all but 2 tablespoons of the soaking water. Combine the soaking water with the remaining ingredients in a small bowl. Grill the chicken, turning as needed and basting twice during cooking with the sauce, for about 20 minutes, or until cooked through.

Per serving
CALORIES: 145 FAT: 2g PROTEIN: 20g CARBOHYDRATES: 10g SODIUM: 211mg CHOLESTEROL: 51mg FIBER: 0.5g

Red Chile—Barbecued Chicken

This sauce is bold and powerful. If you like milder food, cut the red chile powder down to 1½ teaspoons and then taste the sauce, adding more if needed. The sauce can be made the night before, then refrigerated until you grill the chicken the next day.

MAKES 4 SERVINGS

2 tablespoons canola oil

1 small onion, finely chopped

1 garlic clove, minced

1 tablespoon New Mexico red chile powder

1 bay leaf

½ teaspoon grated fresh ginger

½ teaspoon curry powder

¼ teaspoon ground black pepper

1 teaspoon dry mustard (see note, page 68)

1 teaspoon dried thyme

¼ teaspoon crushed red pepper

1 (8-ounce) can tomato sauce

½ cup fresh orange juice

2 tablespoons molasses

1 tablespoon Lea & Perrins Worcestershire
    sauce

1 tablespoon low-sodium, wheat-free tamari
    soy sauce

4 boneless, skinless chicken breast halves

1. Heat the oil in a heavy skillet over medium heat. Add the onion and garlic and sauté over medium-high heat until the onion is transparent. Add the remaining ingredients, except the chicken, and simmer over low heat for about 15 minutes, or until the sauce is reduced to about 1½ cups.

2. Preheat a grill. Rinse the chicken with cold water and pat dry with paper towels. Grill the chicken, turning once and brushing frequently with the sauce for about 20 minutes, or until cooked through.

Per serving

CALORIES: 240 FAT: 9g PROTEIN: 22g CARBOHYDRATES: 19g SODIUM: 726mg CHOLESTEROL: 51mg FIBER: 2g

■ ■ ■

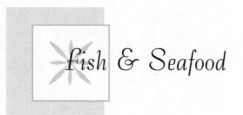

Fish & Seafood

*f*ish is a great component of gluten-free diets because there are so many varieties of fish and there are so many ways to prepare it, ranging from traditional to contemporary.

There are a variety of cooking methods in these recipes, from grilling to roasting to baking in parchment paper at high temperatures for short periods of time. You're sure to find several dishes to add to your repertoire.

Cod Baked with Vegetables

Prepare this dish the night before, refrigerate, then bake when you get home from work. Fix the side dishes while it cooks. You'll be ready for dinner in about thirty minutes.

MAKES 4 SERVINGS

4 (about 4 ounces each) cod or sole fillets

1 tablespoon olive oil

$\frac{1}{3}$ cup diced, peeled carrot

$\frac{1}{3}$ cup finely chopped celery

$\frac{1}{3}$ cup chopped green onions

1 small garlic clove, minced

$\frac{1}{2}$ teaspoon celery salt

$\frac{1}{4}$ teaspoon lemon pepper

$\frac{1}{2}$ teaspoon dried rosemary

1 large tomato, seeded and chopped

1 tablespoon chopped fresh parsley

$\frac{1}{2}$ teaspoon grated lemon zest

2 tablespoons grated Parmesan cheese
   (cow or soy)

1. Preheat the oven to 350°F. Grease an 11 x 7-inch baking dish. Arrange the fish in a single layer in the prepared dish. Set aside.

2. Heat the oil in a skillet over medium heat. Add the carrot, celery, green onions, and garlic and sauté for about 3 minutes. Stir in the celery salt, lemon pepper, rosemary, tomato, parsley, and lemon zest.

3. Spoon the mixture over the fish. Sprinkle with the Parmesan cheese. Bake for 20 to 25 minutes, or until the fish flakes easily.

Per serving
CALORIES: 155 FAT: 5g PROTEIN: 22g CARBOHYDRATES: 5g SODIUM: 348mg CHOLESTEROL: 51mg FIBER: 1g

▪ ▪ ▪

Halibut with Papaya Salsa

The colors in the salsa are absolutely beautiful, and the jalapeño chile adds a little heat. This dish makes a wonderful summertime dinner entrée, but we like it so much that I prepare it year-round.

MAKES 4 SERVINGS; 2 CUPS SALSA

1 ripe papaya

$\frac{1}{4}$ cup finely chopped red bell pepper

$\frac{1}{4}$ cup finely chopped yellow bell pepper

$\frac{1}{4}$ cup finely chopped red onion

2 tablespoons fresh lime juice

$\frac{1}{4}$ cup frozen apple juice concentrate, thawed

$\frac{1}{2}$ teaspoon minced garlic

$\frac{1}{4}$ cup chopped fresh cilantro

1 jalapeño chile, $\frac{1}{8}$ inch cut off stem end and
   seeds removed

$\frac{1}{4}$ teaspoon salt

$\frac{1}{8}$ teaspoon ground white pepper

4 (about 6 ounces each) halibut steaks

1. Peel and finely chop the papaya. Combine all the ingredients, except the fish, in a medium bowl. Cover and refrigerate for up to 4 hours. Remove the chile before serving.

2. Preheat a grill or broiler. Spray the grill rack with cooking spray. Grill the fish for about 10 minutes per side, or until it flakes easily. To serve, top each halibut steak with ½ cup salsa.

Per serving
CALORIES: 280 FAT: 4g PROTEIN: 37g CARBOHYDRATES: 26g SODIUM: 237mg CHOLESTEROL: 54mg FIBER: 2g

▪ ▪ ▪

Orange Roughy in Parchment

*F*ish cooked in parchment comes out very moist, tender, and flavorful. It can be assembled the night before, then baked while you prepare the remainder of the meal. It also makes a wonderful dish for company, because cutting open the parchment paper just before you serve it adds a bit of drama.

MAKES 4 SERVINGS

¼ cup chopped sun-dried tomatoes in oil
¼ cup fresh lemon juice
½ teaspoon grated lemon zest
2 teaspoons dried rosemary
1 small garlic clove, minced
¼ cup chopped green onions
½ teaspoon lemon pepper
½ teaspoon salt
4 (about 6 ounces each) orange roughy fillets

1. Cut 4 (13-inch) parchment paper squares (see note, below). Preheat the oven to 425°F.

2. Combine all the ingredients, except the fish, in a small bowl.

3. Arrange the parchment squares on the countertop. Place one fish fillet in the center of each square. Top with an equal amount of the tomato mixture. Fold the parchment paper over the fish, crimping or folding the edges attractively. Twist the ends tightly to seal. Spray with cooking spray.

4. Place the paper packages on a baking sheet. Bake for about 15 minutes, or until the packages puff up and are lightly browned. Place on individual serving plates. Cut open carefully to avoid steam burns.

Per serving
CALORIES: 160 FAT: 8g PROTEIN: 17g CARBOHYDRATES: 4g SODIUM: 452mg CHOLESTEROL: 23mg FIBER: 0.5g

*N*ote: Aluminum foil can be substituted for the parchment paper. Do not spray with cooking spray.

▪ ▪ ▪

Red Snapper in Parchment

Cooking in parchment produces a flavorful, low-fat dish. The snapper is delightfully seasoned and very colorful.

MAKES 4 SERVINGS

1 tablespoon olive oil

½ cup chopped fresh cilantro

2 medium tomatoes, chopped

2 tablespoons grated onion

1 teaspoon dried rosemary

1 teaspoon dried basil

¼ cup dry white wine

¼ cup black olives, sliced

½ teaspoon grated lemon zest

½ teaspoon salt

¼ teaspoon ground black pepper

4 (about 6 ounces each) red snapper fillets

1. Cut 4 (13-inch) parchment paper squares (see note, page 133). Preheat the oven to 425°F.

2. Combine all the ingredients, except the fish, in a small bowl.

3. Arrange the parchment squares on the countertop. Place one fish fillet in the center of each square. Top with an equal amount of the tomato mixture. Fold the parchment paper over the fish, crimping or folding the edges attractively. Twist the ends tightly to seal. Spray with cooking spray.

4. Place the paper packages on a baking sheet. Bake for about 15 minutes, or until the packages puff up and are lightly browned. Place on individual serving plates. Cut open carefully to avoid steam burns.

Per serving

CALORIES: 290 FAT: 7g PROTEIN: 45g CARBOHYDRATES: 5g SODIUM: 509mg CHOLESTEROL: 81mg FIBER: 1g

■ ■ ■

Salmon and Vegetables in Parchment

This is an easy way to serve salmon and vegetables. Assemble the night before, refrigerate, and then bake while you prepare the remainder of the dinner. This makes an excellent company dish, too. *Julienne* means to cut the vegetables into very thin matchstick-size pieces.

MAKES 4 SERVINGS

½ teaspoon salt

¼ teaspoon ground black pepper

1 teaspoon dried dill weed

1 carrot, peeled and julienned

1 zucchini, julienned

1 red bell pepper, julienned

1 tablespoon grated onion

1 teaspoon grated lemon zest

1 tablespoon olive oil

4 (about 6 ounces each) salmon fillets

1. Cut 4 (13-inch) parchment paper squares (see note, page 133). Preheat the oven to 425°F.

2. Combine all the ingredients, except the fish, in a medium bowl.

3. Arrange the parchment squares on the countertop. Place one fish fillet in the center of each square. Top with an equal amount of the tomato mixture. Fold the parchment paper over the fish, crimping or folding the edges attractively. Twist the ends tightly to seal. Spray with cooking spray.

4. Place the paper packages on a baking sheet. Bake for about 15 minutes, or until the packages puff up and are lightly browned. Place on individual serving plates. Cut open carefully to avoid steam burns.

—————————

Per serving
CALORIES: 245 FAT: 9g PROTEIN: 35g CARBOHYDRATES: 4g SODIUM: 398mg CHOLESTEROL: 88mg FIBER: 1.5g

■ ■ ■

Salmon with Asian Sauce

The light yet slightly spicy sauce is a great companion for salmon.

MAKES 4 SERVINGS

1 cup low-sodium, wheat-free tamari soy sauce

1 tablespoon cornstarch

1 tablespoon peeled grated fresh ginger

1 tablespoon rice vinegar

1 tablespoon olive oil

2 teaspoons honey

¼ teaspoon cayenne pepper

¼ teaspoon ground black pepper

1 garlic clove, minced

4 (about 6 ounces each) salmon fillets

1. Combine all the ingredients, except the fish, in a blender or food processor. Purée until almost smooth.

2. Preheat a grill or broiler. Spray the grill rack with cooking spray. Grill the fish, basting frequently with the sauce, for about 10 minutes per side, or until it flakes easily. Serve immediately.

—————————

Per serving
CALORIES: 280 FAT: 9g PROTEIN: 37g CARBOHYDRATES: 9g SODIUM: 2,048mg CHOLESTEROL: 88mg FIBER: 0.5g

■ ■ ■

Salmon with Maple Glaze

The sweet maple syrup producers a glaze that truly complements the salmon flavor.

MAKES 4 SERVINGS

½ cup fresh lemon juice

¼ cup pure maple syrup

¼ teaspoon maple extract

1 garlic clove, minced

½ teaspoon crushed red pepper

1 teaspoon olive oil

2 tablespoons peeled grated fresh ginger

¼ teaspoon salt

4 (about 6 ounces each) salmon fillets, each
    1 inch thick

1. Combine all the ingredients, except the fish, in a small, heavy saucepan. Simmer over medium heat until the mixture is reduced to about ½ cup. Remove from the heat and cool.

2. Preheat a broiler or grill. Spray the broiler pan with cooking spary. Broil the fish, basting frequently with the sauce, for about 10 minutes per side, or until it flakes easily. Serve immediately.

Per serving

CALORIES 270 FAT: 7g PROTEIN: 34g CARBOHYDRATES: 16g SODIUM: 250mg CHOLESTEROL: 88mg FIBER: 0.5g

■ ■ ■

Red Snapper with Tomato-Lime Salsa

Tomatillos look like green tomatoes, but they're not tomatoes. They produce a slightly tart taste that combines beautifully with the other flavors in this salsa.

MAKES 4 SERVINGS; ABOUT 1 CUP SALSA

2 plum tomatoes, finely chopped

8 medium tomatillos, husks removed and
    chopped

¼ cup finely chopped yellow bell pepper

2 tablespoons finely chopped red onion

1 teaspoon grated lime peel

1 tablespoon fresh lime juice

1 tablespoon honey

¼ teaspoon ground cumin

¼ cup chopped fresh cilantro

1 tablespoon olive oil

4 (about 6 ounces each) red snapper fillets

1. Combine all the ingredients, except the fish, in a medium bowl. Cover and refrigerate for up to 4 hours.

2. Preheat a grill or broiler. Spray the grill rack with cooking spray. Grill the fish for about 10 minutes per side, or until it flakes easily. To serve, top each fillet with ¼ cup of the salsa.

Per serving

CALORIES: 155 FAT: 5g PROTEIN: 18g CARBOHYDRATES: 8g SODIUM: 6mg CHOLESTEROL: 31mg FIBER: 2g

■ ■ ■

Oven-Baked Crab Cakes

Crab cakes are great as appetizers or as a main course. Make bread crumbs from leftover slices of gluten-free Sandwich Bread (page 35)

or French Bread (page 25). Baking rather than frying the crab cakes cuts down on the fat.

MAKES 4 SERVINGS

1 celery stalk, finely chopped

1 tablespoon grated fresh onion

2 large large egg whites

1 tablespoon Durkee shrimp spice

1 tablespoon chopped fresh parsley

¼ teaspoon cayenne pepper

1 tablespoon grated Parmesan cheese
  (cow or soy)

1 tablespoon Lea & Perrins Worcestershire
  sauce

1 teaspoon Italian seasoning

½ cup plain yogurt or ¼ cup milk
  (cow, rice, or soy)

1 tablespoon baking powder

1 cup dried gluten-free bread crumbs

1 pound crabmeat, picked over

1. Preheat the oven to 400°F. Grease a baking sheet or line with parchment paper.

2. Combine all the ingredients, except the bread crumbs and crab, in a medium bowl. Stir in the bread crumbs until thoroughly mixed. Gently stir in the crab. Shape the mixture into 8 crab cakes.

3. Arrange the crab cakes on the prepared baking sheet. Bake for 15 minutes, turn, and bake for 10 minutes longer, or until both sides are lightly browned.

Per serving
CALORIES: 255 FAT: 3g PROTEIN: 30g CARBOHYDRATES: 25g SODIUM: 940mg CHOLESTEROL: 102mg FIBER: 2g

■ ■ ■

Southwestern Crab Cakes

This is a Southwestern version of crab cakes. Serve with the Avocado Chile Sauce (page 82).

MAKES 4 SERVINGS

2 tablespoons plain yogurt or 1½ tablespoons
  milk (cow, rice, or soy)

1 cup shredded Monterey Jack cheese with
  jalapeño or nondairy cheese of choice

½ cup finely minced red bell pepper

½ cup chopped fresh cilantro

1 tablespoon grated onion

1 celery stalk, finely chopped

1 teaspoon Italian seasoning

2 large egg whites

1 cup dried gluten-free bread crumbs

1 pound crabmeat, picked over

1. Preheat the oven to 400°F. Grease a baking sheet or line with parchment paper.

2. Combine all the ingredients, except the bread crumbs and crab, in a medium bowl. Stir in the bread crumbs until thoroughly mixed. Gently stir in the crab. Shape the mixture into 8 crab cakes.

3. Arrange the crab cakes on the prepared baking sheet. Bake for 15 minutes, turn, and bake for 10 minutes longer, or until both sides are lightly browned.

Per serving
CALORIES: 350 FAT: 12g PROTEIN: 36g CARBOHYDRATES: 23g SODIUM: 763mg CHOLESTEROL: 126mg FIBER: 2g

■ ■ ■

Cajun Shrimp on Pasta

This dish has a delightful spiciness, and its colorful display looks so inviting on your plate. You can use purchased gluten-free noodles or your own Homemade Egg Pasta (page 49).

MAKES 6 SERVINGS

1 tablespoon canola oil

8 ounces fresh or frozen snow peas

1 medium red bell pepper, cut into thin strips

1 medium garlic clove, minced

1 tablespoon cornstarch

1 cup low-sodium, gluten-free chicken broth

½ cup dry white wine

½ teaspoon sweet paprika

½ teaspoon dried thyme

½ teaspoon dried basil

¼ teaspoon cayenne pepper

¼ teaspoon ground black pepper

¼ teaspoon crushed red pepper

1 pound medium shrimp, peeled and deveined

1 teaspoon grated lemon zest

1 tablespoon chopped fresh parsley

8 ounces gluten-free pasta

½ cup grated Parmesan cheese (cow or soy), for garnish

1. Heat the oil in a large, heavy skillet over medium heat. Add the snow peas and bell pepper and stir-fry about 3 minutes, or until crisp-tender. With a slotted spoon transfer the vegetables to a bowl and set aside.

2. Add the garlic to the skillet and sauté for 1 minute. Combine the cornstarch and ¼ cup of the broth. Add the cornstarch mixture, remaining ¾ cup broth, and the wine to the garlic and cook, stirring, about 1 minute, or until the sauce thickens. Stir in the paprika, thyme, basil, cayenne, black pepper, and crushed red pepper; bring the mixture to a boil. Add the shrimp, reduce the heat and cook for 5 minutes. Return the vegetables to the skillet and cook for 1 minute longer.

3. Meanwhile, cook the pasta according to package directions.

4. Just before serving, toss the shrimp mixture with the lemon zest and parsley. Serve over hot pasta. Sprinkle with the Parmesan cheese.

Per serving
CALORIES: 290 FAT: 8g PROTEIN: 24g CARBOHYDRATES: 24g SODIUM: 698mg CHOLESTEROL: 159mg FIBER: 2g

■ ■ ■

Crab-Zucchini Casserole

This Italian-flavored dish makes a great lunch or light supper. I like to serve it with crusty French bread and a tossed salad. It's especially good in summer, when fresh tomatoes are in season. You can make your own bread crumbs from leftover French Bread (page 25) or Sandwich Bread (page 35).

MAKES 4 SERVINGS

2 tablespoons olive oil

1 small onion, finely chopped

1 small garlic clove, minced

3 small zucchini, cut crosswise into ⅛-inch-thick slices

3 large tomatoes, seeded and chopped

1⅓ cups diced Swiss cheese or nondairy cheese of choice

1 cup gluten-free bread crumbs, toasted

1 teaspoon salt

1 teaspoon ground black pepper

1 teaspoon dried basil

½ pound crab meat, picked over

½ cup grated Parmesan cheese (cow or soy)

1. Preheat the oven to 375°F. Grease a 2-quart casserole. Heat the oil in a heavy skillet over medium heat. Add the onion and garlic and sauté until the onion is transparent. Add the zucchini and sauté, stirring frequently, for 3 minutes. Remove from the heat.

2. Combine the tomatoes, 1 cup of the Swiss cheese, ¾ cup of the bread crumbs, salt, pepper, and basil in a bowl. Add the onion mixture and crab; mix lightly but thoroughly.

3. Turn the mixture into the prepared casserole. Sprinkle the top with the remaining ¼ cup bread crumbs, ⅓ cup Swiss cheese, and the Parmesan cheese. Bake, uncovered, for 30 to 40 minutes.

Per serving

CALORIES: 375 FAT: 15g PROTEIN: 30g CARBOHYDRATES: 31g SODIUM: 1,321mg CHOLESTEROL: 65mg FIBER: 4g

■ ■ ■

Shrimp Creole

I've been making this recipe for many years and it's still on our list of favorites. The sauce can be made earlier in the day and then reheated just before dinnertime. Add the shrimp just before serving and cook just until they're done.

MAKES 4 SERVINGS

1 tablespoon olive oil

½ cup chopped onion

½ cup chopped celery

1 garlic clove, minced

1 (16-ounce) can tomatoes, undrained

1 (8-ounce) can tomato sauce

1 tablespoon Lea & Perrins Worcestershire
    sauce

1 teaspoon sugar

1 teaspoon salt

½ teaspoon celery salt

¾ teaspoon chile powder

⅛ teaspoon cayenne pepper

2 teaspoons cornstarch mixed with
    1 tablespoon water

1 pound fresh shrimp, peeled and deveined

½ cup chopped green bell pepper

4 cups cooked white rice

¼ cup chopped fresh parsley

1. Heat the oil in a large, heavy Dutch oven over medium heat. Add the onion, celery, and garlic and sauté, stirring occasionally, until tender but not brown. Add the tomatoes, tomato sauce, Worcestershire sauce, sugar, salt, celery salt, chile powder, and cayenne. Simmer, uncovered, for 30 minutes.

2. Stir the cornstarch mixture until blended, then stir it into the tomato sauce. Cook the sauce, stirring constantly, until bubbly. Add the shrimp and bell pepper; cover and simmer for 5 minutes, or until the shrimp are pink. Serve over the rice. Garnish with the parsley.

Per serving

CALORIES: 390 FAT: 5g PROTEIN: 14g CARBOHYDRATES: 72g SODIUM: 1,440mg CHOLESTEROL: 43mg FIBER: 4g

■ ■ ■

Shrimp Curry

This very flavorful curry is guaranteed to tantalize your taste buds.

MAKES 4 SERVINGS

1 teaspoon canola oil

1 large onion, chopped

1 medium red bell pepper, chopped

1 garlic clove, minced

1 tablespoon curry powder

1 teaspoon ground cumin

1 teaspoon ground coriander

¼ teaspoon ground cardamom

1 (12-ounce) can evaporated skim milk or ¾ cup
    milk (cow, rice, or soy)

¼ cup unsweetened coconut milk

1½ pounds shrimp, peeled and deveined

2 tablespoons fresh lime juice

1 tablespoon cornstarch

⅓ cup chopped fresh cilantro

½ teaspoon salt

¼ teaspoon ground black pepper

4 cups cooked white rice

1. Heat the oil in a large, heavy saucepan over medium heat. Add the onion and bell pepper and sauté for about 5 minutes, or until softened. Add the garlic, curry powder, cumin, coriander, and cardamom. Sauté for about 2 minutes, until fragrant. Reduce the heat to low and pour in the milk and coconut

milk. Bring to a simmer, stirring constantly to prevent scorching. Simmer for 5 minutes. Add the shrimp and cook, uncovered, for 10 to 12 minutes, until the shrimp are pink and curled.

2. In a small bowl, combine the lime juice and cornstarch, stirring until smooth. Add to the shrimp mixture and cook, stirring constantly, until thickened. Stir in the cilantro, salt, and pepper. Serve over cooked rice.

Per serving
CALORIES: 595 FAT: 9g PROTEIN: 48g CARBOHYDRATES: 80g SODIUM: 760mg CHOLESTEROL: 260mg FIBER: 4g

■ ■ ■

White Clam Sauce with Linguine

This sauce is wonderful served over linguini, either the purchased version or your own homemade pasta (page 49). It's also good with purchased spinach noodles.

MAKES 4 SERVINGS

2 (15-ounce) cans clams, undrained
¼ cup dry white wine
1 garlic clove, minced
1 teaspoon olive oil
¼ teaspoon dry mustard (see note, page 68)
⅛ teaspoon ground ginger
½ teaspoon onion salt
¼ teaspoon ground white pepper
1 teaspoon instant chopped onion
1 cup milk (cow, rice, or soy)
1 tablespoon cornstarch
2 tablespoons fresh lemon juice
¼ cup chopped fresh parsley
2 cups gluten-free noodles or penne pasta, cooked
¼ cup grated Parmesan cheese (cow or soy)
Sweet paprika, for garnish

1. In a large, heavy saucepan over medium heat, combine the clams with their juices, wine, garlic, and oil and simmer for 5 minutes, until the liquid is slightly reduced. Stir in the mustard, ginger, onion salt, pepper, and onion and cook for 3 minutes.

2. In a small bowl, combine ¼ cup of the milk and the cornstarch, stirring until smooth. Add to the clam mixture with the remaining ¾ cup milk. Cook over medium-low heat, stirring constantly, until the mixture thickens.

3. Remove from the heat and stir in the lemon juice and parsley. Serve over the noodles. Sprinkle with the Parmesan cheese and paprika.

Per serving
CALORIES: 415 FAT: 10g PROTEIN: 12g CARBOHYDRATES: 63g SODIUM: 909mg CHOLESTEROL: 132mg FIBER: 1g

■ ■ ■

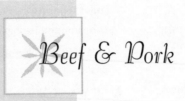

Beef & Pork

Growing up on a farm in Nebraska, I ate plenty of meat and never gave much thought to how it was prepared: fried, baked, roasted, or grilled. When I began a wheat-free diet, I was dismayed to learn how many meat dishes have hidden wheat in them in the form of breading, sauces, gravies, stuffing, and marinades. Now I pay careful attention to how my meat is prepared.

The recipes in this chapter were selected either because they don't require flour at all or because the dish can be prepared using alternatives to wheat flour without sacrificing quality and taste.

Beef Paprikás with Pasta

This is similar to the Hungarian dish, Chicken Paprikás (page 118), but with beef instead. It makes a wonderful, hearty dinner on cold winter nights.

MAKES 4 SERVINGS

1 tablespoon olive oil

1 large onion, chopped

1 pound beef tenderloin, cut into ½-inch cubes

½ cup chopped green bell pepper

1 pound fresh mushrooms, trimmed and sliced

2 cups low-sodium, gluten-free beef broth

1 tablespoon tomato paste

1 tablespoon sweet Hungarian paprika

2 tablespoons cornstarch

2 teaspoons dried dill weed

2 tablespoons white wine

½ cup gluten-free sour cream or sour cream alternative

½ teaspoon celery salt

¼ teaspoon ground black pepper

2 cups cooked purchased gluten-free pasta (noodles or penne) or Homemade Egg Pasta (page 49)

4 tablespoons chopped fresh parsley

1. Heat the oil in a heavy Dutch oven over medium heat. Add the onion, meat, and bell pepper and sauté for about 10 minutes, or until the vegetables are tender and the meat is browned. Add the mushrooms and sauté for 2 to 3 minutes.

2. Stir in 1¾ cups of the broth, the tomato paste, and paprika and simmer, covered, for 8 to 10 minutes.

3. In a small bowl, combine the remaining ¼ cup broth and the cornstarch, stirring until smooth, then stir the mixture into the sauce. Cook, stirring for 3 to 5 minutes, until the sauce thickens.

4. Stir in the dill, wine, sour cream, celery salt, and pepper. (You may have to use a handheld immersion blender to make sour cream alternative blend in.) Heat to serving temperature but do not boil. Serve over the noodles. Garnish with the parsley.

Per serving
CALORIES: 520 FAT: 32g PROTEIN: 33g CARBOHYDRATES: 29g SODIUM: 766mg CHOLESTEROL: 108mg FIBER: 3g

■ ■ ■

Beef Burgundy

This is a favorite company dish at our house, and it's the dish my grown son always requests when he visits.

MAKES 6 SERVINGS

1 bacon slice

2 pounds beef sirloin steak, cut into 1-inch cubes

2 cups chopped onion

4 medium carrots, peeled and cut into
  1-inch pieces

1 small garlic clove, minced

1 teaspoon brandy extract

3 cups burgundy wine

1 ½ cups low-sodium, gluten-free beef broth

2 teaspoons salt

¼ teaspoon ground black pepper

2 tablespoons tomato paste

2 bay leaves

1 teaspoon dried thyme

1 pound mushrooms, trimmed and halved

2 cups fresh or frozen peeled small white
  pearl onions

1 tablespoon cornstarch mixed with
  2 tablespoons water

2 cups cooked purchased gluten-free pasta
  (noodles or penne) or Homemade Egg Pasta
  (page 49), cut into noodles

½ cup chopped fresh parsley

1. Preheat the oven to 325°F. Sauté the bacon in a large, heavy Dutch oven over medium heat until crisp. With a slotted spoon, transfer to a paper towel to drain.

2. Add the meat and chopped onions to the bacon drippings and sauté, stirring occasionally, for about 5 minutes. Add the carrots and garlic; sauté for 2 minutes. Crumble the bacon and add with the brandy extract, wine, broth, salt, pepper, tomato paste, bay leaves, thyme, mushrooms, and pearl onions to the pot. Stir thoroughly and bring to a boil. Cover

and bake for 1 hour, or until the meat is very tender.

3. To thicken the cooking liquid, place Dutch oven over medium heat. Stir in cornstarch mixture until blended, then stir it into the liquid and cook, stirring, until thickened. Serve over the pasta. Sprinkle with the parsley.

Per serving
CALORIES: 450 FAT: 21g PROTEIN: 28g CARBOHYDRATES: 19g SODIUM: 1,160mg CHOLESTEROL: 92mg FIBER: 3g

■ ■ ■

Beef Stroganoff

The rich, creamy texture of this dish suggests it contains lots of fat. However, when made with Yogurt Cheese (page 94), the amount of fat is substantially reduced, without any loss of flavor or creamy texture. You may use a sour cream alternative, if you wish.

MAKES 4 SERVINGS

2 tablespoons canola oil

1 pound beef sirloin steak, cut into
  ½-inch cubes

1 (4-ounce) can mushrooms, drained

½ cup chopped onion

1 small garlic clove, minced

½ teaspoon salt

¼ teaspoon ground black pepper

2 tablespoons tomato paste

2 tablespoons dry white wine

1 (10.5-ounce) can low-sodium beef broth

1 1/2 tablespoons cornstarch

1 cup gluten-free sour cream, sour cream alternative, or Yogurt Cheese (page 94)

2 cups cooked purchased gluten-free pasta (noodles or penne) or Homemade Egg Pasta (page 49), cut into noodles

2 tablespoons chopped fresh parsley

1. Heat the oil in a large, heavy skillet over medium heat. Add the meat and brown quickly on all sides. Add the mushrooms, onion, garlic, salt, and pepper. Cook, stirring occasionally, for about 5 minutes, until the onion is crisp-tender. With a slotted spoon, transfer the mixture to a plate.

2. Add the tomato paste, wine, and 3/4 cup of the broth to the skillet; cook over medium heat, stirring and scraping all the browned bits from the bottom of the skillet.

3. Combine the cornstarch and the remaining 1/4 cup of broth in a small bowl and stir until blended. Stir the cornstarch into the tomato mixture and cook, stirring constantly, until the mixture is thickened and bubbly.

4. Return the meat mixture to the skillet. Reduce the heat to low and stir in the sour cream. (You may have to use a handheld immersion blender to make sour cream alternatives blend in.) Heat to serving temperature but do not boil. Serve over the pasta. Sprinkle with the parsley.

Per serving
CALORIES: 445 FAT: 21g PROTEIN: 30g CARBOHYDRATES: 25g SODIUM: 640mg CHOLESTEROL: 105mg FIBER: 1g

■ ■ ■

Best-Ever Meat Loaf

This makes a very flavorful loaf. Even my gluten-free friends use this recipe. The sauce on top and inside the meat loaf adds extra moisture. Make your own bread crumbs from leftover gluten-free breads. You may use all beef in this recipe if you wish, but the fat content may be higher.

MAKES 4 SERVINGS

1 (8-ounce) can tomato sauce

1/4 cup packed light brown sugar

1/2 teaspoon dry mustard (see note, page 68)

1/2 teaspoon chile powder

1/4 teaspoon ground cloves

1 garlic clove, minced

1 teaspoon Lea & Perrins Worcestershire sauce

3/4 pound lean ground beef

1/4 pound lean ground turkey

1 large egg, lightly beaten

1 cup dried gluten-free bread crumbs

1/2 teaspoon salt

1/4 teaspoon ground black pepper

1 tablespoon instant chopped onion

1. Preheat the oven to 350°F. In a small bowl, combine the tomato sauce, sugar, mustard, chile powder, cloves, garlic, and Worcestershire sauce. Mix well.

2. Add half of the tomato mixture to a large bowl. Add all the remaining ingredients. Mix well with your hands. Shape the mixture into a loaf, either rounded or rectangular, and place in a baking pan. (If desired, place loaf on a metal rack; I use a round, perforated rack, which allows the fat to drip through to the bottom of the pan and keeps the fat away from the loaf during baking.) Make an indentation in the center of the loaf and pour the remaining tomato mixture into this indentation. Bake for 45 minutes, or until the loaf is nicely browned.

Per serving
CALORIES: 430 FAT: 20g PROTEIN: 26g CARBOHYDRATES: 34g SODIUM: 918mg CHOLESTEROL: 134mg FIBER: 3g

■ ■ ■

Mexican Beef Pie

This is a good dish for casual entertaining. It looks pretty, it's inviting, and it tastes great. You may use nondairy Cheddar and Monterey Jack cheeses, if you wish. Guacamole and sour cream can be used as additional garnishes.

MAKES 6 SERVINGS

½ pound lean ground beef
1 cup chopped onion
1 garlic clove, minced
1 tablespoon chile powder
½ teaspoon ground cumin
½ teaspoon ground oregano
¼ teaspoon ground black pepper
⅛ teaspoon ground cinnamon
⅛ teaspoon ground cloves
¼ teaspoon salt
1 teaspoon sugar
1 cup canned tomatoes, undrained
½ cup chopped fresh cilantro
1 (4-ounce) can diced green chiles, undrained
1 (8-ounce) package low-salt corn
　tortilla chips
2 cups cooked or canned pinto beans
1 cup black olives, sliced
½ cup shredded Cheddar cheese
1 cup shredded Monterey Jack cheese
¼ cup chopped green onions, for garnish

1. Preheat the oven to 400°F. In a large, cast-iron skillet or other ovenproof pan, brown the meat and onion over medium heat, stirring to break up the meat. Add the garlic and cook for 1 minute. Stir in the spices, salt, and sugar and cook for 2 minutes to blend flavors. Stir in the tomatoes with their juice, cilantro, and chiles. Reduce the heat to low and simmer, stirring occasionally, for 10 minutes.

2. Transfer the mixture to a large bowl. Wipe the skillet clean with paper towels and coat with cooking spray.

3. Place half of the tortilla chips on the bottom of the skillet. Spoon half of the meat sauce over the chips. Top with half of the beans and all of the olives. Sprinkle with half of the cheeses. Top with the remaining chips and spread the remaining meat sauce on top. Add the remaining 1 cup beans and sprinkle with the remaining cheeses. As the mixture is assembled, use a spatula to press down on the chips. Bake for 20 minutes, or until the mixture is bubbly and the cheeses are browned. Garnish with the green onions.

Per serving

CALORIES: 590 FAT: 34g PROTEIN: 23g CARBOHYDRATES: 50g SODIUM: 890mg CHOLESTEROL: 59mg FIBER: 11g

■ ■ ■

Pizza

This crispy pizza crust tastes so delicious that it has received national acclaim. Use any topping you like along with the delicious fat-free Pizza Sauce (page 89).

MAKES A 12-INCH CRUST; 6 SERVINGS

1 tablespoon active dry yeast
²⁄₃ cup brown rice flour or garbanzo/fava
    bean flour
¹⁄₃ cup tapioca flour
2 tablespoons dry milk powder or nondairy
    milk powder

1 teaspoon xanthan gum
1 teaspoon guar gum
¹⁄₂ teaspoon salt
1 teaspoon unflavored gelatin powder
1 teaspoon Italian seasoning
²⁄₃ cup warm water (110°F)
¹⁄₂ teaspoon sugar
1 teaspoon olive oil
1 teaspoon cider vinegar
Pizza Sauce (page 89) or favorite sauce
Pizza toppings

1. Preheat the oven to 425°F. Spray a 12-inch nonstick pizza pan with cooking spray.

2. In a medium bowl using a mixer with regular beaters (not dough hooks), blend the yeast, flours, dry milk powder, xanthan and guar gums, salt, gelatin, and Italian seasoning on low speed. Add the water, sugar, oil, and vinegar. Beat on high speed for 1 minute. (If the beaters bounce around in the bowl, the dough is too stiff. Add water if necessary, 1 tablespoon at a time, until the dough does not resist the beaters.) The dough should be soft. (You may mix all ingredients together in a food processor for easier blending.)

3. Place the dough on the prepared pizza pan. Liberally sprinkle the dough with rice flour, then press the dough into the pan with your hands, continuing to sprinkle dough with flour to prevent it from sticking to your hands. Make the edge thicker to contain the toppings.

4. Bake the crust for 10 minutes. Remove from the oven. Spread the crust with sauce

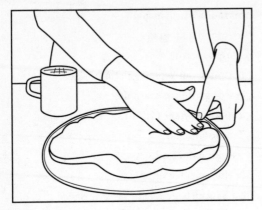

Pizza

and toppings. Bake for 20 to 25 minutes longer, or until the top is nicely browned.

⅛ **of crust:**
CALORIES: 145 FAT: 2g PROTEIN: 4g CARBOHYDRATES: 32g SODIUM: 285mg CHOLESTEROL: 0mg FIBER: 2g

■ ■ ■

Sloppy Joes

One of the first foods I missed on a gluten-free diet was my sloppy joes because the purchased seasoning mix I ordinarily used contained wheat. You can make this easy version the night before; reheat for a quick supper. Use the Hamburger Buns on page 26.

MAKES 4 SERVINGS

1 pound lean ground beef round
1 small onion, finely chopped

1 teaspoon cornstarch
½ teaspoon sugar
1 teaspoon celery salt
1 (6-ounce) can tomato paste
½ teaspoon dry mustard (see note, page 68)
¼ teaspoon garlic powder
¼ teaspoon chile powder
¼ teaspoon dried thyme
⅛ teaspoon ground cloves
1 teaspoon Lea & Perrins Worcestershire sauce
1¼ cups water

1. Brown the meat and onion in a heavy skillet over medium heat, stirring to break up the meat. Drain off the fat and extra juices.

2. Mix the cornstarch and sugar in a small bowl and add to the skillet along with the remaining ingredients and simmer for 10 to 15 minutes.

Per serving
CALORIES: 320 FAT: 20g PROTEIN: 23g CARBOHYDRATES: 11g SODIUM: 654mg CHOLESTEROL: 78mg FIBER: 3g

■ ■ ■

Stir-Fried Ginger Beef with Rice

This is a tasty, colorful Chinese dish that's fun to prepare while your guests watch. For a real group effort, they can help chop the vegetables.

MAKES 4 SERVINGS

2 tablespoons low-sodium, wheat-free tamari
  soy sauce

1 teaspoon sesame oil

2 garlic cloves, minced

1 ½ teaspoons light brown sugar

½ teaspoon crushed red pepper

1 pound lean beef sirloin steak, cut into
  thin strips

3 tablespoons peanut oil

1 cup fresh mushrooms, trimmed and halved

3 tablespoons diced, peeled fresh ginger

1 small onion, chopped

1 pound broccoli florets

1 red bell pepper, cut into thin strips

2 teaspoons cornstarch mixed wtih ¼ cup water

1 cup water

4 cups cooked white rice

1. In a medium bowl, combine 1 tablespoon of the soy sauce with the sesame oil, garlic, brown sugar, and crushed red pepper. Add the meat and marinate at room temperature for 15 minutes.

2. Heat 1 tablespoon of the peanut oil in a large, heavy skillet or wok over high heat. Add the mushrooms and ginger and stir-fry for about 1 minute.

3. Add another 1 tablespoon of peanut oil, the onion, the meat and marinade and stir-fry over medium heat for about 2 minutes, or until the meat is just browned. Transfer the meat and onion to a plate.

4. Return the skillet to high heat and add the remaining 1 tablespoon peanut oil and remaining 1 tablespoon soy sauce. Add the broccoli and bell pepper and stir-fry for 1 minute.

5. Stir the cornstarch mixture until well blended, then stir the cornstarch mixture and the water into the broccoli mixture. Cook, stirring constantly, until thickened.

6. Return the meat and onions to the skillet and heat to serving temperature. Serve over the rice.

Per serving

CALORIES: 600 FAT: 11g PROTEIN: 36g CARBOHYDRATES: 86g SODIUM: 918mg CHOLESTEROL: 66mg FIBER: 6g

■ ■ ■

*T*ostadas

*T*ostadas are fun, easy, and delicious. You can vary the toppings as you wish. You may use nondairy Cheddar and Monterey Jack cheese. Guacamole and sour cream are additional topping options.

MAKES 4 SERVINGS

3 tablespoons canola oil

8 Corn Tortillas (page 42) or use purchased
  6-inch-size gluten-free tostada shells

½ pound ground beef or chicken, cut into
  ½-inch cubes

1 (4-ounce) can diced green chiles, drained

2 small plum tomatoes, diced

2 cups shredded lettuce

1 cup shredded Monterey Jack cheese

½ cup shredded Cheddar cheese

1 cup purchased gluten-free tomato salsa,
    warmed

1. Preheat the oven to 250°F. Heat the oil in a heavy skillet over medium heat. Fry the tortillas, one at a time, for 20 to 40 seconds on each side, until crisp and golden. Drain on paper towels, wrap in foil, and keep warm in oven. (If you're using purchased tostado shells, skip this step.)

2. Drain the excess oil from the skillet. Add the meat and cook over medium heat, stirring to break up the meat, until browned. Stir in the chiles; heat until hot.

3. Top each tortilla with layers in this order: meat, tomatoes, lettuce, and cheeses. Top with the salsa.

Beef Tostadas

Per serving
CALORIES: 600 FAT: 42g PROTEIN: 25g CARBOHYDRATES: 33g SODIUM: 553mg CHOLESTEROL: 88mg FIBER: 5g

Chicken Tostadas

Per serving
CALORIES: 490 FAT: 28g PROTEIN: 29g CARBOHYDRATES: 33g SODIUM: 555mg CHOLESTEROL: 74mg FIBER: 5g

■ ■ ■

Pork Chops in Mushroom Sauce

The pork chops rest in a creamy, onion-flavored mushroom sauce. Served with cooked white rice, this also makes a wonderful company dish. Garnish the platter with bright red cherry tomatoes for color.

MAKES 4 SERVINGS

4 center-cut pork chops (about 1 pound),
    trimmed

1 tablespoon canola oil

1 cup sliced fresh mushrooms

1 tablespoon grated fresh onion

1 small garlic clove, minced

¼ teaspoon salt

¼ teaspoon dried sage

¼ teaspoon white pepper

½ cup dry white wine

½ cup low-sodium, gluten-free chicken broth

1 teaspoon cornstarch mixed with
    1 tablespoon water

½ cup gluten-free sour cream or sour cream
    alternative

2 tablespoons chopped fresh parsley, for garnish

1. Rinse the pork with cold water and pat dry with paper towels.

2. Heat the oil in a heavy skillet over medium heat. Add the pork and fry, turning

once, for about 10 minutes, or until browned. Transfer the chops to a plate and set aside.

3. Add the mushrooms to the skillet and sauté until lightly browned. Stir in the onion, garlic, salt, sage, and pepper. Add the wine and broth. Return the pork to the pan, cover, and simmer for 20 minutes.

4. Stir the cornstarch mixture until well blended, then slowly stir it into the juices around the pork and cook, stirring until the mixture thickens slightly. Stir in the sour cream and heat gently to serving temperature but do not boil. (If you use a sour cream alternative you may have to whisk it into the mixture or use a handheld immersion blender to fully incorporate it.) Garnish with the parsley.

Per serving

CALORIES: 360 FAT: 24g PROTEIN: 26g CARBOHYDRATES: 4g SODIUM: 277mg CHOLESTEROL: 86mg FIBER: 0.5g

■ ■ ■

Pork Chops with Dried Fruit

The flavors of dried fruit complement pork. This dish is especially good in the winter when dried fruits are more commonly eaten.

MAKES 4 SERVINGS

4 center-cut pork chops (about 1 pound), trimmed
Salt and ground black pepper
2 tablespoons canola oil
1 small onion, chopped
2½ cups low-sodium gluten-free chicken broth
¾ cup dry red wine
½ teaspoon dried thyme
½ cup chopped dried plums
¼ cup dried cranberries or dried apricots
¼ teaspoon salt
¼ tablespoon black pepper
4 tablespoons chopped fresh parsley

1. Rinse the pork with cold water and pat dry with paper towels. Season to taste with salt and pepper.

2. Heat the oil in a heavy Dutch oven over medium heat. Add the pork and fry, turning once for about 10 minutes, or until browned. Transfer the chops to a plate and set aside. Add the onion to the Dutch oven and sauté for about 5 minutes, or until browned.

3. Return the pork to the Dutch oven; add the broth, wine, thyme, plums, and cranberries. Bring to a simmer, cover, and cook for about 30 minutes.

4. Using a slotted spoon, transfer the pork chops to a platter. Using the same spoon, transfer the fruit to top of pork; keep warm.

5. Bring the remaining cooking liquid to a boil; boil, stirring occasionally, for 15 to 20 minutes, until thickened slightly. Add ¼ teaspoon each salt and pepper. Spoon the sauce over the pork and sprinkle with the parsley.

Per serving

CALORIES: 400 FAT: 18g PROTEIN: 25g CARBOHYDRATES: 28g SODIUM: 648mg CHOLESTEROL: 56mg FIBER: 2g

■ ■ ■

Pork Chops with Mustard Sauce

This is a quick, easy dish to prepare and the maple-rosemary sauce packs a bold flavor.

MAKES 4 SERVINGS

1 teaspoon olive oil

1 large onion, chopped

4 center-cut pork chops (about 1 pound), trimmed

2 tablespoons Dijonnaise mustard

1 tablespoon pure maple syrup

½ teaspoon dried rosemary

½ teaspoon dried thyme

¼ teaspoon salt

¼ teaspoon ground black pepper

2 tablespoons cider vinegar

4 tablespoons chopped fresh parsley

1. Heat the oil in a large, heavy skillet over medium heat. Add the onion and sauté for 8 to 10 minutes, until slightly transparent. Push the onion to one side of the skillet.

2. Rinse the pork with cold water and pat dry with paper towels. Add the pork to skil-let alongside the onionis, and fry, turning once, for about 10 minutes, or until browned.

3. In a small bowl, stir the mustard, maple syrup, rosemary, thyme, salt, pepper, and vinegar until blended. Add the mixture to the skillet and bring to a boil. Boil, stirring, until the mixture is slightly reduced. Transfer the pork to a serving platter; drizzle with remaining sauce. Sprinkle with the parsley.

Per serving

CALORIES: 215 FAT: 12g PROTEIN: 18g CARBOHYDRATES: 6g SODIUM: 415mg CHOLESTEROL: 56mg FIBER: 1g

■ ■ ■

Pork Tenderloin with Brandy Sauce

This makes a wonderful fall or winter dinner entrée and is especially good as a company dish; my guests always love it. Pork tenderloin is easy to work with because there is no bone and no waste.

MAKES 4 SERVINGS

1 (1¼-pound) pork tenderloin

1 tablespoon ground black pepper

½ cup low-sodium, gluten-free chicken broth

1 tablespoon grated fresh onion

½ teaspoon dried thyme leaves

1 teaspoon brandy extract

¼ cup plain yogurt or 2 tablespoons milk (cow, rice, or soy)

2 tablespoons butter or margarine
(see note, page 23)
1 tablespoon fresh lemon juice
¼ teaspoon salt
¼ teaspoon ground white pepper
¼ cup chopped fresh chives or parsley

1. Preheat the oven to 400°F. Rinse the tenderloin and pat dry with paper towels. Rub the tenderloin with the black pepper. Place on a rack in a shallow baking pan and roast for about 20 minutes, or until a meat thermometer registers 155°F when inserted in the thickest part of the meat. Remove from the oven, cover with foil, and let stand for 10 minutes.

2. Meanwhile, combine the broth and onion in a medium saucepan and bring to a boil over medium heat. Reduce the heat, cover, and simmer for 2 minutes. Add the thyme and brandy extract and simmer, uncovered, over medium heat for 5 minutes.

3. Reduce the heat to low. Whisk in the yogurt. Add the butter, 1 tablespoon at a time, stirring constantly with a wire whisk, until blended. Stir in the lemon juice, salt, and white pepper.

4. To serve, cut the tenderloin into 1-inch-thick slices. Place 3 slices on each plate; top with sauce. Sprinkle with the chives.

Per serving

CALORIES: 275 FAT: 11g PROTEIN: 32g CARBOHYDRATES: 3g SODIUM: 316mg CHOLESTEROL: 108mg FIBER: 0.5g

■ ■ ■

Pork Tenderloin with Apple Chutney

The chutney that accompanies this dish is spectacular, and the aroma that fills your kitchen is heavenly. It is always enthusiastically endorsed by my holiday guests.

MAKES 4 SERVINGS

¼ cup olive oil
4 garlic cloves, minced
1 teaspoon dried thyme leaves
4 teaspoons ground cumin
2 teaspoons cayenne pepper
1 teaspoon ground cinnamon
1 (1¼-pound) pork tenderloin
Salt and black pepper, to taste
1 cup Apple Chutney (page 93)

1. Combine the oil, garlic, thyme, cumin, cayenne, and cinnamon in a small bowl. Rub the spice mixture over the pork. Cover and refrigerate for at least 4 hours or overnight.

2. Preheat the oven to 400°F. Season the pork with salt and pepper. In a large nonstick skillet, brown the pork on all sides.

3. Transfer the pork to a large baking pan and roast for about 20 minutes, or until a meat thermometer inserted in the thickest part of the meat registers 155°F. Remove the pork from the oven, cover with foil, and let

stand for 10 minutes. Cut the pork into ½- to ¾-inch-thick slices. Serve with the chutney.

_____

Per serving
CALORIES: 355 FAT: 19g PROTEIN: 30g CARBOHYDRATES: 15g SODIUM: 194mg CHOLESTEROL: 92mg FIBER: 1.5g

■ ■ ■

Pork with Apples and Cabbage

This is a very easy, very rustic casserole that goes great with a crusty, hearty bread, such as Fennel (page 29) or Pumpernickel (page 30).

MAKES 4 SERVINGS

1 pound pork loin, cut into 1-inch cubes

1 tablespoon olive oil

1½ teaspoons dried rosemary, crushed

½ cup chopped onion

2 cups coarsely chopped cabbage

1 apple, peeled, cored, and chopped

½ cup dry white wine

½ cup apple juice

½ teaspoon celery salt

1. Rinse the pork with cold water and pat dry with paper towels. Heat the oil in a large, heavy skillet over medium heat. Add the pork, rosemary, and onion and sauté, stirring occasionally, for about 5 minutes, or until the pork is deeply browned on all sides.

2. Add the remaining ingredients and bring to a boil. Cover, reduce the heat, and simmer, stirring occasionally, for 30 minutes.

_____

Per serving
CALORIES: 240 FAT: 11g PROTEIN: 18g CARBOHYDRATES: 11g SODIUM: 251mg CHOLESTEROL: 56mg FIBER: 1g

■ ■ ■

Spareribs with Chile Glaze

This glaze is slightly spicy due to the combination of both chile and chile powders. The addition of maple syrup and orange juice further complements this spicy glaze and helps to moderate its spiciness.

MAKES 4 SERVINGS

4 pounds pork spareribs

½ cup fresh orange juice

¼ cup olive oil

2 tablespoons pure maple syrup

1 garlic clove, minced

2 teaspoons dried oregano

1½ teaspoons New Mexico red chile powder
   (see headnote, page 99)

1½ teaspoons chile powder

1 teaspoon celery salt

1. Preheat the oven to 350°F. Spray a large roasting pan with cooking spray. Rinse the spareribs with cold water and pat dry with paper towels. Arrange, meaty side down, on a metal rack in the prepared pan.

2. Combine the remaining ingredients in a small bowl. Spread over both sides of the spareribs. Bake for 30 minutes. Turn and bake for 30 minutes longer, or until the ribs are browned and cooked through. (If you wish, you can grill the spareribs instead, basting them frequently with the glaze.) Slice between the ribs and serve.

Per serving

CALORIES: 885 FAT: 70g PROTEIN: 48g CARBOHYDRATES: 12g SODIUM: 634mg CHOLESTEROL: 220mg FIBER: 1g

■ ■ ■

Sweet-and-Sour Pork

This has been a family favorite for the past twenty years. I often make it when I have left-over vegetables in my refrigerator.

MAKES 4 SERVINGS

3 tablespoons low-sodium, wheat-free tamari
   soy sauce
1 teaspoon ground ginger
1 tablespoon cornstarch
1 garlic clove, minced

1 (8-ounce) can pineapple chunks in juice,
   undrained
1 pound boneless lean pork, cut into 1-inch cubes
1 tablespoon canola oil
1 small onion, diced
1 medium carrot, peeled and cut into 1/4-inch-
   thick rounds
1 small green bell pepper, chopped
1/2 cup chopped red bell pepper
2 tablespoons light brown sugar
3 tablespoons cider vinegar
2 tablespoons low-sodium, wheat-free tamari
   soy sauce
1 tablespoon grated, peeled fresh ginger
1/8 teaspooon white pepper
1 tablespoon cornstarch mixed with
   2 tablespoons water
4 cups cooked white rice

1. Combine 1 tablespoon of the soy sauce, ground ginger, cornstarch, garlic, and 1 tablespoon of the pineapple juice in a medium bowl. Rinse the pork with cold water and pat dry with paper towels. Add the pork and marinate for about 15 minutes.

2. Heat the oil in a heavy skillet over medium heat. Add the onion, carrot, and pork and sauté, stirring frequently, until lightly browned. With a slotted spoon, transfer the pork, onion, and carrot to a medium bowl; set aside. Add the bell peppers and sauté over medium heat, stirring frequently, for 3 minutes. Transfer the peppers to a small bowl; set aside.

3. Add the pineapple (including the remaining juice and enough water to equal ⅔ cup liquid), brown sugar, vinegar, remaining 2 tablespoons soy sauce, fresh ginger, and white pepper to the skillet. Stir the cornstarch mixture and slowly stir it into the pineapple mixture. Cook, stirring constantly, until the mixture thickens slightly.

4. Return the pork mixture to the skillet. Cover and simmer for 10 minutes. Add the bell peppers and heat to serving temperature. Serve over the rice.

Per serving
CALORIES: 505 FAT: 4g PROTEIN: 11g CARBOHYDRATES: 105g SODIUM: 773mg CHOLESTEROL: 5mg FIBER: 7g

■ ■ ■

Thai Pork Noodle Bowl

You can find this dish in Thai or Vietnamese restaurants, but it's really easy to make at home. It's fun to eat and very colorful.

MAKES 4 SERVINGS

1 tablespoon canola oil

½ pound boneless, lean pork, cut into
 ½-inch cubes

¼ cup chopped green onions

1 garlic clove, minced

½ cup chopped red bell pepper

¼ cup gluten-free rice vinegar

3 tablespoons low-sodium, wheat-free tamari
 soy sauce

6 tablespoons packed light brown sugar

4 teaspoons sweet paprika

1 teaspoon Reese anchovy paste

¾ teaspoon cayenne pepper

1 cup chopped fresh cilantro

1 (12-ounce) package purchased rice noodles,
 cooked and drained

2 cups mung bean sprouts

¼ cup chopped peanuts or cashews, for garnish

1. Heat the oil in a large, heavy skillet over medium heat. Add the pork, green onions, and garlic and sauté, stirring occasionally, until the pork is lightly browned and cooked through. Add the bell pepper and cook for 1 minute.

2. Meanwhile, in a small bowl, combine the vinegar, soy sauce, brown sugar, paprika, anchovy paste, and cayenne. Add to the pork mixture and toss to combine. Stir in the cilantro and cook until heated through.

3. Divide the noodles among 6 individual serving bowls. Top with the pork mixture and bean sprouts. Garnish with the peanuts.

Per serving
CALORIES: 400 FAT: 13g PROTEIN: 17g CARBOHYDRATES: 55g SODIUM: 278mg CHOLESTEROL: 74mg FIBER: 4g

■ ■ ■

Baked Ham with Wine Sauce

This makes a wonderful Easter entrée or the main dish for a special Sunday dinner.

MAKES 10 SERVINGS; ABOUT 2 CUPS SAUCE

1 (5-pound) fully cooked ham

2 cups low-sodium, gluten-free chicken broth

½ cup red wine

1 bay leaf

¼ cup orange juice concentrate

½ teaspoon dried thyme

⅛ teaspoon ground cloves

1 cup golden raisins

1 tablespoon cornstarch mixed with
  2 tablespoons water

1. Preheat the oven to 325°F. Place the ham in a heavy roasting pan. Bake for 1 hour, or until heated through.

2. Meanwhile, in a medium, heavy saucepan, combine the broth, wine, bay leaf, orange juice concentrate, thyme, and cloves. Bring to a boil, then remove from the heat and cool. Add the raisins.

3. When ready to serve, return the sauce to medium heat. Cook for about 10 minutes, or until the sauce is slightly reduced.

4. Stir the cornstarch mixture until well blended, then stir it into the sauce. Cook, stirring constantly, until the mixture thickens slightly. Slice the ham and serve with the sauce.

Per serving

CALORIES: 600 FAT: 30g PROTEIN: 51g CARBOHYDRATES: 26g SODIUM: 3,938mg CHOLESTEROL: 162mg FIBER: 1g

■ ■ ■

Chorizo

Chorizo is a traditional hot and spicy Mexican sausage, so a little goes a long way. Although sausage is typically a high-fat item, you can control the fat content by grinding your own lean meat rather than buying it already ground. I often just brown the sausage meat without shaping it into links or patties if I'm in a hurry.

MAKES 12 TO 16 SAUSAGES

1 pound ground beef round

2 pounds ground lean pork

1 tablespoon sweet paprika

⅓ cup cider vinegar

1 teaspoon salt

1 teaspoon crushed red pepper

2 teaspoons dried oregano

3 garlic cloves, minced

1 teaspoon ground coriander

1 teaspoon ground cumin

½ teaspoon ground cloves

1. In a large bowl, mix the meats together by hand. Add the remaining ingredients. Mix thoroughly, using a spatula or your hands. Shape into a large ball or log, cover, and refrigerate for at least 4 hours.

2. Shape the meat mixture into patties, about ½ inch thick and 2 inches in diameter. (If you prefer link sausage, shape into links about 3 inches long and ¾ inch in diameter.)

3. Coat a nonstick pan with cooking spray. Add the sausages and fry over medium heat until nicely browned on both sides. Transfer to paper towels to drain. You can freeze the cooked sausages for up to 2 weeks.

Per sausage

CALORIES: 320 FAT: 22g PROTEIN: 26g CARBOHYDRATES: 1g SODIUM: 259mg CHOLESTEROL: 97mg FIBER: 0.5g

■ ■ ■

Country Sausage

Now you can enjoy sausage, knowing that there's no wheat flour or bread filler. This version excludes unnecessary fat. If you grind your own meat, you can really control the fat content. If you'd like, you can brown the sausage meat without shaping it into links or patties.

MAKES 12 SAUSAGES

1 pound ground beef round

1 pound ground lean pork

1 pound ground turkey

4 garlic cloves, minced

6 green onions, minced

½ cup *each* finely chopped green and red
  bell peppers

2 teaspoons chopped fresh cilantro

2 teaspoons ground cumin

2 teaspoons dried thyme

2 teaspoons fennel seeds

¼ teaspoon ground nutmeg

½ teaspoon crushed red pepper

1 teaspoon salt

1. In a large bowl, mix the meats together by hand. Add the remaining ingredients. Mix thoroughly, using a spatula or your hands. Shape into a large ball or log, cover, and refrigerate for at least 4 hours.

2. Shape the meat mixture into patties, about ½ inch thick and 2 inches in diameter. (If you prefer link sausage, shape into links about 3 inches long and ¾ inch in diameter.)

3. Coat a nonstick pan with cooking spray. Add the sausages and fry over medium heat until nicely browned on both sides. Transfer to paper towels to drain. You can freeze the cooked sausages for up to 2 weeks.

Per sausage

CALORIES: 290 FAT: 17g PROTEIN: 25g CARBOHYDRATES: 7g SODIUM: 279mg CHOLESTEROL: 92mg FIBER: 2g

■ ■ ■

Spaghetti and Meatballs

This dish has been a family favorite for years. I reduce the fat by browning the meatballs in the oven rather than in a skillet. Be sure to use lean beef and pork, or use some ground turkey to further cut the fat. The meatballs freeze well for up to one month.

MAKES 12 SERVINGS

1 pound ground beef round
¼ pound ground lean pork
½ teaspoon salt
½ teaspoon ground black pepper
½ cup dried gluten-free bread crumbs
2 large eggs
3 tablespoons dried parsley
1 tablespoon dried basil
1 teaspoon dried oregano
1 garlic clove, minced
3 tablespoons grated Romano cheese
½ teaspoon crushed red pepper flakes
Spaghetti Sauce (page 88)
6 cups cooked purchased, gluten-free spaghetti
   or Homemade Egg Pasta (page 49)

1. Preheat the oven to 350°F. Combine all the ingredients, except the sauce and pasta, in a large bowl and mix well. Shape into 1½-inch balls and place on a baking sheet. Bake for 20 minutes, or until browned. Remove from the oven and cool on the baking sheet for 15 minutes.

2. Add the meatballs to the sauce. Heat to serving temperature. Serve over the spaghetti.

―――――――――

Per serving
CALORIES: 575 FAT: 20g PROTEIN: 22g CARBOHYDRATES: 77g SODIUM: 1,406mg CHOLESTEROL: 170mg FIBER: 4g

■ ■ ■

Swedish Meatballs

So easy to make and so wonderful to eat. You can brown the meatballs the night before and make the sauce when you get home from work. You'll have a meal in less than thirty minutes. Make your own bread crumbs from leftover gluten-free Sandwich Bread (page 35) or French Bread (page 25). Serve the hot meatballs over cooked white rice, mashed potatoes, gluten-free pasta, or Wild Rice Pancakes (page 64).

MAKES 4 SERVINGS

MEATBALLS
½ pound ground round
½ pound ground pork
¼ cup dry gluten-free bread crumbs
1 small onion, finely chopped
1 large egg, slightly beaten
2 garlic cloves, minced

½ teaspoon ground allspice

¼ teaspoon ground nutmeg

½ teaspoon salt

¼ teaspoon ground black pepper

SAUCE

1 tablespoon cornstarch

1 cup low-sodium gluten-free beef broth

4½ teaspoons dried dill weed

1 cup gluten-free sour cream or sour cream
    alternative

1 tablespoon brandy extract

1. Preheat the oven to 350°F. Coat a baking sheet with cooking spray. To make the meatballs: Combine all the ingredients in a medium bowl. Shape into 24 (1-inch) meatballs.

2. Place the meatballs on the prepared baking sheet. Bake for 20 minutes, or until browned.

3. To make the sauce: Mix the cornstarch with 3 tablespoons of the broth in a small bowl. Heat the remaining broth and 1 teaspoon of the dill in a large saucepan over medium heat. Add the cornstarch mixture and cook, stirring constantly, until thickened.

4. Add the meatballs to the sauce and simmer for 10 minutes. Stir in the sour cream and brandy extract. (If you're using a sour cream alternative, you have to whisk it into some of the sauce first to fully incorporate it.) Sprinkle with the remaining dill.

Per serving
CALORIES: 390 FAT: 23g PROTEIN: 33g CARBOHYDRATES: 10g SODIUM: 602mg CHOLESTEROL: 147mg FIBER: 0.5g

■ ■ ■

Lasagne

You can enjoy lasagne, when it's made with gluten-free pasta. You can make your own pasta (page 49) or purchase the variety found in health food stores. If you use fresh pasta, you don't have to cook it first. This recipe is dairy based.

MAKES 10 SERVINGS

½ pound ground beef round

1 pound low-fat ricotta cheese

½ cup low-fat cottage cheese

½ cup grated Parmesan cheese (cow or soy)

1 large egg, slightly beaten

2 cups Spaghetti Sauce (page 88)

1 pound low-fat mozzarella cheese,
    shredded (4 cups)

12 gluten-free lasagne noodles, cooked

1. Preheat the oven to 350°F. Grease a 13 x 9-inch baking pan. Cook the beef in a medium skillet over medium heat, stirring to break up the meat, until browned. Drain off any fat; set aside.

2. Combine the ricotta, cottage, and Parmesan cheeses and the egg in a medium bowl. Mix well.

3. Reserve ¾ cup of the sauce and 1 cup of the mozzarella cheese for the top of the lasagne. Spread ½ cup of the sauce on the bottom of the prepared pan. Arrange 4 lasagne noodles over the sauce. Spread half of the ricotta mixture over the noodles, then half of the meat, then 1½ cups of the mozzarella cheese and half of the sauce. Repeat the layers, ending with noodles. Top with the reserved ¾ cup sauce and 1 cup mozzarella.

4. Bake for 30 to 40 minutes, or until the cheese has melted and the sauce bubbles around the edge of the pan. Let stand for 10 minutes; cut into squares.

Per serving

CALORIES: 710 FAT: 21g PROTEIN: 39g CARBOHYDRATES: 88g SODIUM: 692mg CHOLESTEROL: 79mg FIBER: 4g

VARIATION

Meatless Lasagne
Omit the ground beef round.

Per serving

CALORIES: 655 FAT: 17g PROTEIN: 35g CARBOHYDRATES: 88g SODIUM: 677mg CHOLESTEROL: 63mg FIBER: 4g

■ ■ ■

White Bean Cassoulet with Sausage

Fix this on a cold winter day when you want a hearty, hot meal but don't want to spend a lot of time in the kitchen. Cook the beans in your slow cooker while you're at work. Assemble the cassoulet when you get home and bake it while you prepare the remainder of the meal.

MAKES 6 SERVINGS

3 cups white beans, picked over and rinsed
6 cups water
1 bay leaf
1 teaspoon salt
½ pound Country Sausage (page 158)
½ pound boneless pork, cut into 1-inch cubes
1 large onion, chopped
2 garlic cloves, minced
1 (28-ounce) can whole tomatoes, drained
⅓ cup chopped fresh parsley
1 teaspoon dried rosemary
1 teaspoon dried thyme
½ teaspoon ground black pepper
½ teaspoon celery salt

1. Combine the beans, water, bay leaf, and salt in a slow cooker. Cook on low for 8 hours or all day. Discard the bay leaf.

2. Preheat the oven to 400°F. Grease 4 individual ovenproof dishes. In a large, heavy ovenproof skillet, brown the sausage meat, pork, onion, and garlic over medium-high heat, stirring to break up the sausage. With a slotted spoon, transfer the meat mixture to paper towels to drain.

3. Combine the meat mixture with the beans and the remaining ingredients in a large bowl. Spoon into the prepared dishes. Cover with foil and bake for 20 minutes. Uncover and bake for 20 minutes longer. Serve hot.

Per serving

CALORIES: 570 FAT: 18g PROTEIN: 36g CARBOHYDRATES: 69g SODIUM: 750mg CHOLESTEROL: 49mg FIBER: 17g

■ ■ ■

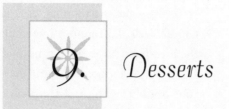

9. Desserts

Walking past a bakery or pastry shop can be absolute torture for the gluten-free crowd. The heavenly aromas stimulate our senses, yet we can't indulge our fondness for cakes, cookies, pastries, and all those other decadent delicacies. Of course, in today's weight-conscious society, desserts are also off-limits for other reasons as well. But it's no fun to avoid dessert, especially when those around you are enjoying it. In this chapter, you'll find a tempting array of sweets specially designed for you! They're so delicious your family and friends won't even notice they're gluten-free.

While this is not a low-fat, low-calorie cookbook, much of the fat and sugar have been removed from the recipes in this section. There's even an Easy Chocolate Cheesecake that has only 225 calories per serving and only three grams of fat.

Enjoy these desserts. Think of them as your reward for committing to and sticking with a gluten-free diet.

Cherry Cobbler

Fruit cobblers are such a treat, nestled under a rich, biscuit blanket. Top with frozen yogurt or ice cream, if you wish, or just drizzle heavy cream over the top for true decadence.

MAKES 6 SERVINGS

FILLING

4 cups pitted tart red cherries or other fresh
    fruit such as apricots, blackberries, peaches,
    or nectarines

½ cup sugar

1 tablespoon quick-cooking tapioca

1 teaspoon grated lemon zest

1 tablespoon fresh lemon juice

1 teaspoon vanilla extract

TOPPING

1 cup flour blend (page 11)

½ cup sugar, plus 1 teaspoon for sprinkling

⅓ cup milk (cow, rice, or soy)

¼ cup margarine (see note, page 23),
    at room temperature

1 large egg

1 tablespoon fresh lemon juice

1 teaspoon grated lemon zest

1 teaspoon baking powder

1 teaspoon vanilla extract

½ teaspoon xanthan gum

¼ teaspoon salt

1. Preheat oven to 375°F. Grease 8-inch-square pan. To make the filling: Combine all the ingredients in the prepared pan and set aside.

2. To make the topping: In a large bowl, combine all the topping ingredients, except the 1 teaspoon sugar, stirring just until blended. Drop by tablespoonfuls onto the fruit mixture. Sprinkle with the 1 teaspoon sugar.

3. Bake for 35 to 40 minutes, or until the filling is bubbly and the crust is golden. Serve warm.

Per serving
CALORIES: 400 FAT: 9g PROTEIN: 4g CARBOHYDRATES: 82g SODIUM: 224mg CHOLESTEROL: 30mg FIBER: 3g

■ ■ ■

Cherry-Apricot Crisp

I find the combination of cherries, dried apricots, and a hint of almond very pleasing to my palate, and the crispy topping adds a nice texture. Be sure to use tart red pie cherries rather than the darker, sweeter Bing cherries.

MAKES 6 SERVINGS

1 pound red tart cherries, pitted and drained

1 (6-ounce) package dried apricots, chopped

¾ cup granulated sugar

2 tablespoons quick-cooking tapioca

½ teaspoon almond extract

2 tablespoons canola oil

½ cup brown rice or sorghum flour

¼ cup packed light brown sugar

¼ teaspoon ground cinnamon

½ teaspoon grated lemon zest

¼ cup sliced almonds

1. Grease an 8-inch-square pan. Combine the cherries, apricots, granulated sugar, tapioca, and almond extract in the prepared pan. Let stand for 30 minutes.

2. Preheat the oven to 375°F. Combine the flour, brown sugar, cinnamon, and lemon zest in a medium bowl. With a pastry blender, cut in the oil until mixture resembles coarse meal. Mix in the almonds. Sprinkle the topping over the fruit, leaving a 1-inch border on all sides.

3. Bake for about 30 minutes, or until the topping is browned. Let cool for 20 minutes before serving.

Per serving

CALORIES: 390 FAT: 9g PROTEIN: 5g CARBOHYDRATES: 80g SODIUM: 9mg CHOLESTEROL: 0mg FIBER: 1g

▪ ▪ ▪

Bananas with Rum Sauce

This dessert is a refreshing change from cake, pie, or cookies, and it is so simple to make. Plus, it provides another serving of fruit to your daily intake.

MAKES 4 SERVINGS

2 teaspoons butter or canola oil

2 tablespoons light brown sugar

2 teaspoons vanilla extract

¼ cup orange juice concentrate, thawed

½ teaspoon ground cinnamon, plus additional for garnish

1 teaspoon rum extract

4 bananas (ripe but not mushy)

1. Combine the butter, brown sugar, vanilla, orange juice concentrate, cinnamon, and rum flavoring in a large, nonstick skillet. Cook over low heat for 1 minute.

2. Peel the bananas. Cut each banana in half crosswise, then lengthwise so there are a total of 4 pieces per banana. Add to the pan and cook for 30 seconds.

3. Arrange 4 banana pieces on each of 4 plates. Spoon the sauce over the bananas and garnish with a sprinkle of cinnamon.

Per serving

CALORIES: 150 FAT: 4g PROTEIN: 1g CARBOHYDRATES: 29g SODIUM: 42mg CHOLESTEROL: 10mg FIBER: 2g

▪ ▪ ▪

Clafouti

Clafouti is French in origin and hard to define; part pudding, part cobbler, part crepe. It is one of the easiest dishes to make. A variety of different fruits will work; try apricots, cherries, or apples instead of peaches. Blueberries and purple-colored fruits such as plums often overpower the delicate topping with their darker colors and abundant juices.

MAKES 4 SERVINGS

¼ cup flour blend (page 11)

½ teaspoon salt

2 large eggs

⅓ cup milk (cow, rice, or soy)

1 teaspoon vanilla extract

½ teaspoon grated lemon zest

2 tablespoons canola oil

3 cups chopped peaches

2 tablespoons powdered sugar

1. Preheat the oven to 375°F. Combine the flour blend, salt, eggs, milk, vanilla, lemon zest, and oil in a blender and blend for 1 minute on high speed (or use a handheld, immersion blender).

2. Grease a 9-inch, ovenproof skillet or 2 small, ovenproof skillets. Place the skillet over medium heat and pour in one-fourth of the batter, spreading it over the bottom of the pan. Cook for 2 to 3 minutes, until the batter resembles a cooked crepe. Remove from the heat.

3. Arrange the fruit on top of the cooked batter. Top with remaining batter. Bake the large skillet for 35 to 40 minutes and small skillets for 20 to 25 minutes, or until the top is puffy and golden brown. Remove from the oven and dust with powdered sugar. Serve immediately.

───────────

Per serving
CALORIES: 225 FAT: 7g PROTEIN: 4g CARBOHYDRATES: 39g SODIUM: 200mg CHOLESTEROL: 163mg FIBER: 2g

■ ■ ■

Carrot Cake

This ever-popular carrot cake derives extra flavor and texture from pineapple, coconut, and nuts. It is always a hit at family gatherings. Omit the frosting if you have dairy sensitivities. Sometimes I just sift lots of powdered sugar on the top, instead.

MAKES 12 SERVINGS

CAKE

2½ cups flour blend (page 11)

2 teaspoons xanthan gum

2 teaspoons baking soda

2 teaspoons ground cinnamon

½ teaspoon ground ginger

1 teaspoon salt

4 large eggs

1 cup packed light brown sugar

1 cup granulated sugar

⅓ cup canola oil

¾ cup milk (cow, rice, or soy)

1 teaspoon vanilla extract

3 cups shredded carrots

1½ cups crushed pineapple, drained
   very well

1 cup shredded coconut

1 cup walnuts, chopped

CREAM CHEESE FROSTING

1 (3-ounce) package nonfat cream cheese,
   softened

2 cups powdered sugar

2 tablespoons milk

1 teaspoon vanilla extract

1. To make the cake: Preheat the oven to 350°F. Grease a 10-cup nonstick Bundt pan. Combine the flour blend, xanthan gum, baking soda, cinnamon, ginger, and salt together in a bowl. Set aside.

2. In a large bowl, combine the eggs, sugars, oil, milk, and vanilla and beat until blended. Beat the flour mixture slowly into the egg mixture until blended. Stir in the carrots, pineapple, coconut, and nuts.

3. Pour the batter into the prepared pan. Bake for 45 to 50 minutes, or until a toothpick inserted in the center of the cake comes out clean. Cool in the pan on a wire rack for 10 minutes. Turn out onto a wire rack and cool completely.

4. To make the frosting: Combine the cream cheese, powdered sugar, milk, and vanilla in a medium bowl. Beat until smooth. Use to frost the cake.

Per serving
CALORIES: 525 FAT: 12g PROTEIN: 6g CARBOHYDRATES: 100g SODIUM: 483mg CHOLESTEROL: 62mg FIBER: 2g

■ ■ ■

Chocolate Cake

This is a small, but very versatile cake. Serve it plain, with a dusting of powdered sugar, or with the optional glaze. Save any leftovers and crumble them into crusts for pies or cheesecakes.

MAKES 12 SERVINGS

CAKE

1¼ cups flour blend (page 11)

½ cup unsweetened cocoa powder
   (not Dutch)

1 teaspoon xanthan gum

1 teaspoon baking soda

¾ teaspoon salt

1 cup packed light brown sugar

2 teaspoons vanilla extract

½ cup milk (cow, rice, or soy)

½ cup butter or margarine (see note, page 23)

1 large egg

¾ cup hot water or brewed coffee

COFFEE GLAZE (Optional)

1/2 cup powdered sugar

2 tablespoons strong brewed coffee

1. Preheat the oven to 350°F. Grease a 9-inch-round or -square nonstick pan or 2 (8-inch-round) pans and line with waxed paper or parchment paper and grease again. The batter can be baked in 12 muffin cups; grease or use paper liners.

2. To make the cake: Combine all the ingredients, except the hot water, in a large bowl and blend with an electric mixer. Add the hot water and mix until thoroughly blended.

3. Pour into prepared pan/s. Bake 9-inch pan for 30 to 35 minutes, 8-inch pans for 25 to 30 minutes, and cupcakes for 20 to 25 minutes, or until a toothpick inserted in center of cake comes out clean. Cool in the pan on a wire rack for 10 minutes. Turn out on wire rack, remove the paper, and cool completely.

4. To make the glaze: Combine the sugar and coffee in a small bowl. Drizzle over the cooled cake, if you like.

Per serving

CALORIES: 200 FAT: 9g PROTEIN: 3g CARBOHYDRATES: 28g
CHOLESTEROL: 38mg SODIUM: 250mg FIBER: 2g

VARIATION

Mexican Chocolate Cake

For a Southwestern adaptation, add 1 1/2 tablespoons almond extract and 1 tablespoon ground cinnamon to the batter in step 2. Bake and cool as instructed. Frost with Chocolate Glaze (page 195).

■ ■ ■

Elegant Dessert Trifle

This dish looks pretty when it's assembled in individual clear glass goblets or in a straight-sided, glass serving dish, which reveal the layers of ingredients to the eye. It's a great way to use up leftover cake. You can vary the fruits for different effects. Strawberries are the most colorful, but kiwifruit, fresh peaches, and blueberries create a stunning appearance as well.

MAKES 6 SERVINGS

6 cups sliced strawberries

1/2 cup orange juice

1 tablespoon powdered sugar

3 cups yogurt (vanilla, lemon, or orange—cow or soy)

Yellow Cake (page 169), cut into 1/2-inch cubes

Whole strawberries, for decoration

1. Combine the sliced strawberries, orange juice, and sugar in a bowl.

2. Layer the ingredients in a glass serving dish, starting with the yogurt, then the cake and sliced strawberries. Repeat the layers, ending with the yogurt. Decorate with the whole berries. Cover and refrigerate for a few hours or overnight. Serve chilled.

Per serving

CALORIES: 225 FAT: 7g PROTEIN: 6g CARBOHYDRATES: 36g SODIUM: 104 mg CHOLESTEROL: 37mg FIBER: 2g

■ ■ ■

Yellow Cake

A good yellow cake is an absolute essential for so many recipes. This one has a hint of lemon. Freeze any leftovers for later use, or keep one in the freezer ready to use.

MAKES 10 SERVINGS

1/3 cup unsalted butter or margarine
   (see note, page 23)

1 cup sugar

2 large eggs, lightly beaten

2 teaspoons grated lemon zest

1 1/2 cups flour blend (page 11)

1 1/2 teaspoons xanthan gum

1/4 teaspoon baking powder

1/4 teaspoon baking soda

1/4 teaspoon salt

3/4 cup buttermilk or 1 tablespoon lemon juice

plus enough milk (cow, rice, or soy) to
   equal 3/4 cup

1 teaspoon vanilla extract

1. Preheat the oven to 325°F. Grease an 11 x 7-inch nonstick pan. Set aside.

2. With an electric mixer on medium speed, beat the butter and sugar in a large bowl until light and fluffy. Reduce the speed to low. Add the eggs and beat until blended. Stir in the lemon zest.

3. Sift the flour blend, xanthan gum, baking powder, baking soda, and salt into a medium bowl. In another medium bowl, combine the buttermilk and vanilla. On low speed, alternately beat the dry ingredients and the buttermilk into the butter mixture, beginning and ending with the dry ingredients. Mix just until combined. Spoon the batter into prepared pan and smooth the top.

4. Bake the cake for 25 to 30 minutes, or until the top is golden brown and a toothpick inserted in the center comes out clean. Cool the cake in the pan on a wire rack for 5 minutes. Turn out onto a wire rack and cool completely. The cake can be wrapped in foil and frozen for 1 month.

Per serving

CALORIES: 280 FAT: 8g PROTEIN: 3g CARBOHYDRATES: 51g SODIUM: 125mg CHOLESTEROL: 54mg FIBER: 0.5g

■ ■ ■

Pineapple Upside-Down Cake

Using the Yellow Cake batter (page 169) makes this family favorite so easy to create. You may use strawberries or raspberries instead of maraschino cherries; add them after the cake has baked.

MAKES 8 SERVINGS

½ cup packed light brown sugar
1 (16-ounce) can pineapple rings in juice, drained (about 7 rings)
7 maraschino cherries, drained
Batter for Yellow Cake (page 169)
Whipping cream, for garnish (optional)

1. Preheat the oven to 350°F. Grease a 10-inch pie plate or cast-iron skillet, or use a special pan designed for upside-down cakes.
2. Evenly sprinkle the sugar over the bottom of the pan. Arrange 7 pineapple slices in a single layer over the sugar. Place a cherry in the center of each ring. Pour the cake batter evenly over the pineapple and cherries.
3. Bake for 35 to 40 minutes, or until the top springs back when touched. Cool in the pan for 5 minutes, then invert onto a serving plate. Garnish with whipped cream, if desired.

Per serving
CALORIES: 355 FAT: 2g PROTEIN: 1g CARBOHYDRATES: 87g
SODIUM: 128mg CHOLESTEROL: 8mg FIBER: 2g

■ ■ ■

Spice Cake

This is a stunningly flavorful cake, an absolute winner that never fails to garner praise. Its spicy flavors marry well with the Seven-Minute Coffee Frosting (page 196).

MAKES 10 SERVINGS

2 cups flour blend (page 11)
1½ teaspoons xanthan gum
1¾ teaspoons baking soda
¾ teaspoon salt
1 tablespoon ground ginger
2 teaspoons ground cinnamon
½ teaspoon ground nutmeg
¼ teaspoon ground cloves
1½ cups milk (cow, rice, or soy)
1½ cups packed light brown sugar
¼ cup butter or margarine (see note, page 23)
¼ cup canola oil
⅓ cup molasses
1 teaspoon vanilla extract
2 large eggs, lightly beaten

1. Preheat the oven to 325°F. Grease a 9-inch-round nonstick pan. Line the bottom with waxed paper, then spray again.

2. Sift the flour blend, xanthan gum, baking soda, salt, and spices into a large bowl.

3. Combine the milk and sugar in a heavy saucepan and bring just to a boil over medium heat. Remove from the heat and add the butter, oil, molasses, and vanilla.

4. When the butter has melted, add the butter mixture to the dry ingredients and mix until thoroughly blended. Add the eggs and mix until blended. Pour the batter into the prepared pan.

5. Bake for 50 minutes, or until a toothpick inserted in the center of the cake comes out clean. Cool the cake in the pan on a wire rack for 5 minutes. Invert the cake onto a plate, remove the paper, and cool completely.

Per serving

CALORIES: 400 FAT: 13g PROTEIN: 4g CARBOHYDRATES: 71g
SODIUM: 468mg CHOLESTEROL: 53mg FIBER: 1g

▪ ▪ ▪

Sponge Cake

This cake, similar to angel food cake but made with whole eggs, not just the whites, is wonderful to serve with fresh fruit, such as strawberries or raspberries.

MAKES 12 SERVINGS

¼ cup fresh lemon juice
1 teaspoon grated lemon zest
9 extra-large eggs
1 cup powdered sugar
¼ cup granulated sugar
1 teaspoon vanilla extract
1 cup potato starch
¼ teaspoon cream of tartar

1. Preheat the oven to 375°F. Mix the lemon juice and lemon zest in a small bowl.

2. Separate 7 of the eggs, being careful not to get any egg yolk in the egg whites. Add the remaining 2 eggs to the egg yolks and beat until foamy and lemon-colored. Gradually beat in the sugars. Mix in the vanilla.

3. Sift the potato starch into the yolk mixture, alternating with the lemon juice and zest. With a mixer on low speed, beat just until blended.

4. Using clean beaters, beat the egg whites until stiff peaks form. Beat in the cream of tartar. Pour the yolk mixture over the egg whites. Use a wire whisk or perforated spoon to carefully and slowly fold the egg whites into the yolk mixture. It's important not to disturb the egg whites too much or the cake will fall.

5. Pour the batter into an ungreased 10-inch tube pan with a removable bottom. Bake in the center of the oven for 30 to 35 minutes. Invert the cake in the pan on a wire rack to cool for 1 hour.

6. Run a thin, sharp knife around the edge of the pan to loosen the cake, then remove the cake from the pan. Using the knife, carefully remove the bottom of the pan from the cake. Place the cake on a platter to serve.

Per serving

CALORIES: 160 FAT: 3g PROTEIN: 4g CARBOHYDRATES: 28g
SODIUM: 40mg CHOLESTEROL: 135mg FIBER: 0g

■ ■ ■

Gingerbread with Lemon Sauce

Dense, moist, and flavorful—this ginger-bread is further enhanced by a piquantly sweet Lemon Sauce.

MAKES 8 SERVINGS

GINGERBREAD

$\frac{1}{2}$ cup packed light brown sugar

$\frac{1}{4}$ cup canola oil

1 large egg

$\frac{1}{2}$ cup molasses

1$\frac{1}{2}$ cups flour blend (page 11)

1 teaspoon xanthan gum

1 teaspoon baking soda

1$\frac{1}{2}$ teaspoons ground ginger

$\frac{3}{4}$ teaspoon ground cinnamon

$\frac{1}{2}$ teaspoon ground cloves

$\frac{1}{2}$ teaspoon salt

$\frac{1}{2}$ cup buttermilk or 1 teaspoon cider vinegar
plus enough milk (cow, rice, or soy) to
equal $\frac{1}{2}$ cup

LEMON SAUCE

$\frac{1}{4}$ cup sugar

1 tablespoon cornstarch

$\frac{1}{8}$ teaspoon salt

$\frac{1}{2}$ cup hot water

2 teaspoons grated lemon zest

1 tablespoon fresh lemon juice

2 teaspoons butter or margarine
(see note, page 23)

1. Preheat the oven to 350°F. Grease an 8- or 9-inch-square nonstick pan.

2. To make the gingerbread: In a large bowl, beat the sugar and canola oil with an electric mixer on medium speed. Beat in the egg, then the molasses and beat well. In another bowl, combine the flour blend, xanthan gum, baking soda, spices, and salt. Add the flour mixture alternately with the buttermilk to the egg mixture.

3. Pour the batter into prepared pan. Bake for 30 minutes, or until a toothpick inserted in the center comes out clean. Cool in the pan on a wire rack.

4. To make the sauce: In a small saucepan, combine the sugar, cornstarch, and salt. Gradually stir in the water. Cook, stirring, over medium heat until the mixture boils and thickens. Stir in the lemon zest, lemon juice, and butter. Serve warm over the gingerbread.

Per serving

CALORIES: 350 FAT: 9g PROTEIN: 3g CARBOHYDRATES: 69g SODIUM: 365mg CHOLESTEROL: 25mg FIBER: 1g

■ ■ ■

Cheesecake

This tastes just like the authentic New York cheesecake, even though I've removed a great deal of the fat and calories by using dry-curd cottage cheese. It tastes great plain, but you can top it with fresh fruit, such as strawberries or blueberries. This recipe contains dairy, so dairy-sensitive folks should avoid it.

MAKES 10 SERVINGS

1 cup crushed Vanilla Wafers (page 182) or
   Pamela's or Enjoy Life cookies
1 cup dry-curd cottage cheese
3 large eggs
2 (8-ounce) packages nonfat cream cheese, at
   room temperature
1 teaspoon grated lemon zest
2 tablespoons fresh lemon juice
1 tablespoon tapioca flour
1 cup sugar
1 1/2 teaspoons vanilla extract
1/4 teaspoon salt

1. Grease the bottom and sides of a 7-inch springform pan. Press the crushed cookies onto the bottom of the pan and slightly up the sides. Chill while preparing the filling.

2. Preheat the oven to 300°F. In a food processor, process the cottage cheese and eggs for 3 minutes, or until the cottage cheese is very, very smooth. Add the remaining ingre-dients and process until very smooth. Slowly pour the filling into the chilled crust.

3. [sic]

4. Bake for 1 hour, or until the cheesecake is set. Let cool in pan on a wire rack. Cover and chill for up to 8 hours or overnight.

5. Release the pan side and remove it; transfer the cheesecake to a serving plate.

Per serving
CALORIES: 275 FAT: 6g PROTEIN: 12g CARBOHYDRATES: 42g
SODIUM: 391mg CHOLESTEROL: 62mg FIBER: 0g

■ ■ ■

Easy Chocolate Cheesecake

My tasters described this dessert as "rich and yummy" even though it contains nonfat cream cheese and low-fat cottage cheese. The crust is made with Chocolate Wafer Cookies (page 176) or any gluten-free chocolate cookies you have on hand. This dessert is quick and easy to make in your food processor. This recipe is dairy-based.

MAKES 8 SERVINGS

1/4 cup crushed Chocolate Wafer Cookies (page
   176) or Pamela's cookies
2 (8-ounce) packages nonfat cream cheese
1 cup (1% fat) cottage cheese
1 cup packed light brown sugar
1/3 cup plus 1 tablespoon unsweetened cocoa
   powder (not Dutch)

½ cup tapioca flour

¼ cup skim milk

1 teaspoon vanilla extract

1 teaspoon chocolate extract (optional)

¼ teaspoon salt

1 large egg

2 tablespoons gluten-free chocolate chips

Fresh fruit, for garnish

1. Preheat the oven to 300°F. Grease the bottom of a 7-inch springform pan. Press the cookies onto bottom of the pan.

2. In a food processor, cream the cream cheese and cottage cheese until very, very smooth. Add the brown sugar, cocoa, flour, milk, vanilla, chocolate extract, if using, and salt. Process until smooth. Add the egg and process just until blended. Stir in the chocolate chips. Slowly pour the mixture over the crumbs in the pan.

3. Bake for 1 hour, or until the cheesecake is set. Let cool in the pan on a wire rack. Cover and chill for at least 8 hours or overnight. Release the pan side and remove it; transfer the cheesecake to a serving plate. Garnish with fresh fruit.

Per serving

CALORIES: 225 FAT: 3g PROTEIN: 13g CARBOHYDRATES: 37g SODIUM: 513mg CHOLESTEROL: 32mg FIBER: 1g

■ ■ ■

Flourless Chocolate Almond Cake

This crowd-pleaser is extremely simple to make. But if you're strapped for time, you can simplify it even further by using the whole eggs without first whipping the whites to soft peaks. The cake won't be as light and airy, but it is still a winner!

MAKES 8 SERVINGS

2 cups slivered almonds

1 cup packed light brown sugar

½ cup canola oil

⅓ cup unsweetened cocoa powder

1 teaspoon almond extract

½ teaspoon salt

4 large eggs, separated

Favorite frosting, melted chocolate, or powdered sugar, for topping

1. Preheat the oven to 350°F. Grease an 8- or 9-inch springform pan. Line the bottom with waxed paper or parchment paper.

2. Grind the nuts in a food processor to a cornmeal-like texture. Add the brown sugar, oil, cocoa, almond extract, salt, and egg yolks and blend until thoroughly mixed.

3. In a large bowl, beat the egg whites with an electric mixer on high speed until soft peaks form. Gently fold the cocoa mixture

into the egg whites, adding one-fourth of the mixture at a time. Transfer the batter to prepared pan.

4. Bake for 40 to 45 minutes, or until a toothpick inserted in the center comes out clean. (The cake rises as it bakes, then falls slightly as it cools.) Cool in the pan on a wire rack for 15 minutes. Run the tip of a thin knife around the edge to loosen the cake from the pan. Release the pan side and remove it; invert the cake onto a serving plate. Remove the paper. Top as desired. Slice the cake into 8 pieces.

Per serving (without topping)

CALORIES: 315 FAT: 24g PROTEIN: 6g CARBOHYDRATES: 23g SODIUM: 169mg CHOLESTEROL: 90mg FIBER: 3g

■ ■ ■

Chocolate Brownies

These brownies are very dense, more like fudge than cake. Serve them plain or with a dusting of powdered sugar, or for a really decadent brownie, top with melted bittersweet chocolate.

MAKES 12 SMALL SERVINGS

1 cup flour blend (page 11)
$^{1}/_{2}$ cup unsweetened cocoa powder (not Dutch)
$^{1}/_{2}$ teaspoon baking powder
$^{1}/_{2}$ teaspoon salt

1 teaspoon xanthan gum
$^{1}/_{3}$ cup margarine (see note, page 23), at room temperature, or canola oil
$^{1}/_{2}$ cup packed light brown sugar
$^{1}/_{2}$ cup granulated sugar
1 large egg
2 teaspoons vanilla extract
$^{1}/_{3}$ cup hot water or brewed coffee
$^{1}/_{2}$ cup chopped walnuts

1. Preheat the oven to 350°F. Grease an 8-inch-square pan.

2. In a large mixing bowl, combine the flour blend, cocoa, baking powder, salt, and xanthan gum; stir until blended. Beat in the margarine, sugars, and egg with an electric mixer on medium speed until well combined. Add the vanilla and water and mix until just blended. Stir in the nuts.

3. Spread the batter evenly in the prepared pan. Bake for 20 minutes, or until a toothpick inserted in the center comes out almost clean. Don't overbake. Cool the brownies before cutting them into 12 pieces.

Per serving

CALORIES: 145 FAT: 5g PROTEIN: 2g CARBOHYDRATES: 25g SODIUM: 128mg CHOLESTEROL: 11mg FIBER: 1g

■ ■ ■

Chocolate Chip Cookies

Everybody's favorite. Now you can enjoy these treats along with everyone else.

MAKES 24 COOKIES

1¼ cups flour blend (page 11)

1 teaspoon xanthan gum

½ teaspoon baking soda

¼ teaspoon salt

¼ cup shortening (see note, page 207) or margarine (see note, page 23), at room temperature, or Spectrum spread

¾ cup packed light brown sugar

⅓ cup granulated sugar

1 teaspoon vanilla extract

1 extra-large egg

1 cup semisweet gluten-free, dairy-free chocolate chips

¼ cup chopped walnuts

1. Preheat the oven to 350°F. Grease a baking sheet or line with parchment paper. Sift the flour blend, xanthan gum, baking soda, and salt into a bowl. Set aside.

2. In a large bowl, with an electric mixer on medium speed, beat the shortening and sugars until blended. Beat in the vanilla and egg, scraping the sides of the bowl frequently. Reduce the speed to low. Beat in the flour mixture until thoroughly mixed. (Or blend all the ingredients together in a food processor.) Stir in the chocolate chips and nuts.

3. Drop the dough by tablespoonfuls on the prepared baking sheet. (If you use Spectrum spread, the cookies may not spread; flatten them slightly with a spatula before baking.)

4. Bake in the center of the oven for 10 minutes. (For chocolate chip bars, bake the dough in an 8-inch-square pan for 25 to 30 minutes.) Cool for 2 to 3 minutes before removing the cookies from the baking sheet. Finish cooling the cookies on a wire rack.

Per cookie
CALORIES: 100 FAT: 4g PROTEIN: 1g CARBOHYDRATES: 16g SODIUM: 75mg CHOLESTEROL: 8mg FIBER: 0.5g

◼ ◼ ◼

Chocolate Wafer Cookies

Use these cookies just as you would use the purchased kind, either as a treat by themselves, or crush them into crumb crusts for pies and cheesecakes. I keep a batch in the freezer, then make them into crumbs with my food processor.

MAKES 24 COOKIES

¼ cup butter or margarine (see note, page 23), at room temperature

2 tablespoons honey

½ cup packed light brown sugar

1 large egg

1 teaspoon vanilla extract

1⅓ cups flour blend (page 11)

¼ cup unsweetened cocoa powder (not Dutch)

1½ teaspoons baking powder

½ teaspoon xanthan gum

½ teaspoon salt

1. In a large bowl, beat the butter, honey, sugar, egg, and vanilla until blended.

2. In another bowl, combine the flour blend, cocoa, baking powder, xanthan gum, and salt. Stir the dry ingredients into the egg mixture to make a dough. Shape the dough into a soft ball. Cover and refrigerate for 1 hour.

3. Preheat the oven to 325°F. Grease a baking sheet or line with parchment paper.

4. Dust your hands with cocoa powder or spray with cooking spray. Shape the dough into 1-inch balls. Place the balls on the prepared baking sheet. Flatten slightly with the bottom of a glass dipped into cocoa powder or sprayed with cooking spray. Bake for 25 to 30 minutes, or until the cookies appear dry on top. Cool for 2 to 3 minutes before removing the cookies from the baking sheet. Finish cooling the cookies on a wire rack.

Per 2 cookies

CALORIES: 170 FAT: 5g PROTEIN: 2g CARBOHYDRATES: 32g SODIUM: 192mg CHOLESTEROL: 25mg FIBER: 1g

■ ■ ■

Coconut Macaroons

This is a very moist, chewy macaroon. Topping the macaroons with chocolate makes them even more delectable. You can dip one end of each cookie into melted chocolate or just drizzle it lightly over them.

MAKES 15 COOKIES

1 (14-ounce) package sweetened shredded coconut

1 cup powdered sugar

½ cup potato starch

1 teaspoon xanthan gum

⅛ teaspoon salt

3 egg whites

1 teaspoon vanilla extract

1. Preheat the oven to 350°F. Grease a large baking sheet or line with parchment paper. Set aside.

2. Combine the coconut, sugar, potato starch, xanthan gum, and salt in a food processor and pulse just until blended. Add the egg whites and vanilla and process until completely mixed. The dough will be stiff.

3. With wet hands, form the dough into 15 (1½-inch) balls and place at least 1 inch apart on the prepared baking sheet.

4. Bake for 15 to 20 minutes or until the cookies start to brown around the edges. Re-

move from the oven and cool on the baking sheet on a wire rack for 10 minutes. Transfer to the wire rack and cool completely. Store in an airtight container.

Per cookie

CALORIES: 225 FAT: 11g PROTEIN: 2g CARBOHYDRATES: 33g SODIUM: 121mg CHOLESTEROL: 0mg FIBER: 1g

■ ■ ■

Biscotti

Biscotti are especially great to keep on hand for a quick snack with your coffee or tea. They travel very well; I've taken them to Europe with great success!

MAKES 30 COOKIES

1 ½ cups slivered almonds

2 cups flour blend (page 11)

¾ cup sugar

1 ½ teaspoons xanthan gum

1 teaspoon baking powder

¼ teaspoon salt

½ cup unsalted butter or margarine (see note, page 23), at room temperature

2 large eggs

¼ cup corn syrup

½ teaspoon vanilla extract

½ teaspoon almond extract

1. Preheat the oven to 350°F. Grease a nonstick baking sheet or line with parchment paper.

2. Process the almonds in a food processor until finely ground. Add the flour blend, sugar, xanthan gum, baking powder, and salt and pulse on and off until mixed. Add the remaining ingredients and pulse the food processor on and off about 20 times or until the ingredients are moist. Then process continuously until the mixture forms a ball, scraping down the sides of the bowl if necessary.

3. Form the dough into a ball. Divide the dough in half. Shape each half into a 2-inch-wide, ½-inch-thick, 12-inch-long log. Place the logs on the prepared baking sheet.

4. Bake for 20 to 25 minutes, or until the logs are browned at the edges. Cool on the baking sheet for 5 minutes. Leave the oven on. With a serrated knife or electric knife, cut each log on the diagonal into ¾-inch-thick slices. Arrange the slices, cut sides down, on the baking sheet.

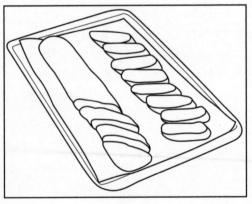

Biscotti

5. Bake for 10 to 15 minutes, or until the biscotti start to brown, turning the slices over halfway during baking to brown both sides. Transfer to a wire rack to cool.

Per cookie

CALORIES: 155 FAT: 8g PROTEIN: 2g CARBOHYDRATES: 22g SODIUM: 38mg CHOLESTEROL: 21 mg FIBER: .05g

■ ■ ■

Granola Bars

Commercially prepared granola bars can be very high in sugar and fat, and they often contain ingredients we can't eat. These bars are great for a quick, nutritious snack, and they travel well.

MAKES 12 BARS

2 cups long-grain brown rice

4 cups water

½ teaspoon salt

1 teaspoon vanilla extract

½ cup dried apricot halves

½ cup shelled sunflower seeds

¼ cup packed light brown sugar

2 tablespoons canola oil

2 cups canned peaches, drained

½ cup unsweetened flaked coconut

½ cup golden raisins

1. Bring the rice and water to a boil in a medium, heavy saucepan over high heat. Reduce the heat to low, cover, and simmer for 30 to 45 minutes, until the rice is tender. Cool.

2. Preheat the oven to 300°F. Grease a 13 x 9-inch nonstick pan. In a food processor, in two batches, combine the rice with the remaining ingredients, except the coconut and raisins, and purée until smooth. Transfer to a bowl and stir in the coconut and raisins.

3. Spread the mixture evenly in the prepared pan. Bake for 1 hour. Remove from the oven and cut into 12 bars. Bake for another 20 minutes, or until the top is lightly browned. Cool on a wire rack. Wrap individual bars in plastic wrap or aluminum foil. Refrigerate for up to 1 week or freeze for 1 month.

Per bar

CALORIES: 180 FAT: 7g PROTEIN: 3g CARBOHYDRATES: 30g SODIUM: 105mg CHOLESTEROL: 0mg FIBER: 2g

■ ■ ■

Apricot Rum Balls

Keep these on hand for unexpected guests. They're especially nice at the holidays, because they keep well and can be dressed up by rolling them in a little powdered sugar.

MAKES 24 BALLS

²/₃ cup slivered almonds

2 cups dried apricots

²/₃ cup powdered sugar

¹/₄ cup light or dark rum

¹/₂ teaspoon vanilla extract

2 teaspoons grated orange zest

3 ounces bittersweet chocolate, finely grated

1. In a food processor, process the almonds until very finely chopped. Add the apricots and pulse until they are finely chopped. Transfer to a medium bowl.

2. Stir in the sugar, rum, vanilla, orange zest, and chocolate. Roll into 24 (1-inch) balls. Refrigerate for up to 1 week in an airtight container.

———————

Per ball

CALORIES: 80 FAT: 2g PROTEIN: 1g CARBOHYDRATES: 16g SODIUM: 2mg CHOLESTEROL: 0mg FIBER: 0.5g

■ ■ ■

Mexican Wedding Cakes

In the Southwest where I live, these little morsels are quite common, especially during the holidays. Store them in a cool place.

MAKES 36 COOKIES

1 cup margarine (see note, page 23), at room temperature

1 cup powdered sugar, plus extra for rolling

2¹/₂ cups flour blend (page 11)

1¹/₂ teaspoons xanthan gum

¹/₃ cup finely chopped pecans

1 teaspoon vanilla extract

¹/₂ teaspoon salt

1. Combine all the ingredients in a food processor, and blend until the mixture forms a ball. Shape into a flat disk, cover, and refrigerate for 2 hours.

2. Grease a baking sheet or line with parchment paper. Form the dough into 36 (1¹/₂-inch) balls. Place on the prepared baking sheet and refrigerate for 30 minutes.

3. Preheat the oven to 350°F. Bake the cookies for 10 to 15 minutes, or until set. Roll in powdered sugar to coat while warm.

———————

Per cookie

CALORIES: 125 FAT: 6g PROTEIN: 1g CARBOHYDRATES: 18g SODIUM: 90mg CHOLESTEROL: 0mg FIBER: 0.5g

■ ■ ■

Gingersnaps

These cookies are great for snacking at home, but they also travel very well. Keep some in your freezer to make crumb crusts for pies.

MAKES 16 COOKIES

¹/₄ cup butter or margarine (see note, page 23), at room temperature

3 tablespoons molasses

½ cup packed light brown sugar

1 teaspoon vanilla extract

1½ cups flour blend (page 11)

1 teaspoon xanthan gum

1 teaspoon baking soda

½ teaspoon salt

1½ teaspoons ground ginger

1½ teaspoons ground cinnamon

¼ teaspoon ground nutmeg

¼ teaspoon ground cloves

2 tablespoons water, if needed

1 tablespoon granulated sugar, for rolling

1. In a large bowl, beat the butter, molasses, brown sugar, and vanilla until blended.

2. In another bowl, combine the flour blend, xanthan gum, baking soda, salt, and spices. Stir the dry ingredients into the butter mixture, adding water if necessary to form a dough that can be shaped into a soft ball. (Or blend all the ingredients, except the granulated sugar, in a food processor.) Cover and refrigerate for 1 hour.

3. Preheat the oven to 325°F. Grease a baking sheet or line with parchment paper.

4. Dust your hands with rice flour and shape the dough into 16 (1-inch) balls. Roll each ball in granulated sugar and place on the prepared baking sheet. Flatten the balls slightly with the bottom of a drinking glass that has been dipped in sugar or sprayed with cooking spray.

5. Bake the cookies for 20 to 25 minutes, or until they start to brown on the bottoms.

Cool the cookies on the baking sheet on a wire rack for about 5 minutes, then transfer them to the wire rack to cool completely. Store in airtight containers.

Per cookie

CALORIES: 135 FAT: 3g PROTEIN: 1g CARBOHYDRATES: 27g SODIUM: 178mg CHOLESTEROL: 8mg FIBER: 0.5g

■ ■ ■

Lemon Bars

This is one of my favorite desserts. For best results, bake these the day before so they have time to firm up.

MAKES 12 BARS

CRUST

1 cup flour blend (page 11)

¼ cup margarine (see note, page 23), chilled

¼ cup powdered sugar

1 teaspoon xanthan gum

¼ teaspoon salt

FILLING

1½ cups powdered sugar, plus extra
    for dusting

¾ cup flour blend (page 11)

½ teaspoon xanthan gum

2 large eggs

3 large egg yolks

¼ cup fresh lemon juice

1 tablespoon grated lemon zest

¼ teaspoon salt

1. Preheat the oven to 350°F. Grease an 8-inch-square pan.

2. To make the crust: In a food processor, combine all the ingredients and process until crumbly. Press the mixture on the bottom of the prepared pan, using plastic wrap to prevent it from sticking to your fingers. Bake for 10 to 15 minutes, or until slightly dry looking. Cool slightly. Leave oven on.

3. To make the filling: In the same food processor, combine all the ingredients and process until the mixture thickens. Pour over the crust. Bake for 20 to 25 minutes, or until set. Cool in the pan on a wire rack. Cut into 12 bars. Dust with powdered sugar.

Per bar

CALORIES: 250 FAT: 6g PROTEIN: 3g CARBOHYDRATES: 47g SODIUM: 120mg CHOLESTEROL: 93mg FIBER: 0.5g

■ ■ ■

Vanilla Wafers

These little cookies taste great and they're indispensable. They travel well, they make great crumb crusts for pies, and they can be crumbled into a crisp topping for puddings and fruit desserts.

MAKES 16 TO 20 COOKIES

¼ cup margarine (see note, page 23), at room temperature

2 tablespoons honey

½ cup packed light brown sugar

2 teaspoons vanilla extract

1½ cups flour blend (page 11)

½ teaspoon xanthan gum

½ teaspoon salt

¾ teaspoon baking soda

1 teaspoon cider vinegar

2 tablespoons water, if needed

1. In a food processor, combine all the ingredients and process until the mixture forms a ball, adding water only if necessary to form a ball. Cover the ball tightly and refrigerate for 1 hour.

2. Preheat the oven to 325°F. Grease a baking sheet or line with parchment paper.

3. With rice-floured hands, shape the dough into 1-inch balls and place on the prepared baking sheet. Bake for 15 to 20 minutes, or until lightly browned. Remove them from the cookie sheet and cool completely on a wire rack.

Per cookie

CALORIES: 128 FAT: 3g PROTEIN: 1g CARBOHYDRATES: 25g SODIUM: 161mg CHOLESTEROL: 0mg FIBER: 0.5g

VARIATION

Anise–Pine Nut Cookies
Add 1 to 2 teaspoons anise flavoring and ¼ cup finely chopped, toasted pine nuts in step 1. Bake as directed.

■ ■ ■

Vanilla Cream Pie

Cream pies are delicious and rich-tasting, yet they're often thickened with wheat flour. Now, you can enjoy them using these recipes.

MAKES 6 SERVINGS

Vanilla Custard (page 193)
1 (9-inch) Crumb Crust for Pies (page 185) or Baked Single Crust (page 187)

Spoon the custard into the baked crust. Cover and refrigerate until well chilled before cutting.

Per serving
CALORIES: 415 FAT: 23g PROTEIN: 5g CARBOHYDRATES: 48g SODIUM: 239mg CHOLESTEROL: 98mg FIBER: 0.5g

VARIATIONS

Banana Cream Pie
Slice 2 bananas into prepared Crumb Crust for Pies. Spoon the custard over the bananas. Cover and re-

frigerate until chilled before cutting. To serve, top each slice with 1 tablespoon whipped cream, if desired. Makes 6 servings

Per serving
CALORIES: 435 FAT: 23g PROTEIN: 6g CARBOHYDRATES: 54g SODIUM: 239mg CHOLESTEROL: 98mg FIBER: 1g

Coconut Cream Meringue Pie
Stir 1 cup sweetened, flaked coconut into the custard. Spoon the custard into the Crumb Crust for Pies. Top with meringue made from 2 egg whites beaten until stiff with 2 tablespoons sugar. Sprinkle with 2 tablespoons sweetened, flaked coconut. Bake in a preheated 425°F oven for 5 to 10 minutes, or until the meringue is nicely browned. Refrigerate until chilled before cutting. Garnish with toasted coconut, if desired. Makes 6 servings

Per serving
CALORIES: 500 FAT: 27g PROTEIN: 7g CARBOHYDRATES: 59g SODIUM: 292mg CHOLESTEROL: 98mg FIBER: 1g

■ ■ ■

Boston Cream Pie

If you don't want to cut the cake layer in half, bake the batter in 2 (8-inch-round) cake pans.

MAKES 10 SERVINGS

Yellow Cake (page 169), baked in 8-inch-round cake pan

Vanilla Custard (page 193)

Chocolate Glaze (page 195)

1. Cool the cake and slice horizontally into 2 layers. Place the bottom layer, cut side up, on a serving plate. Top with the custard and place the top layer, cut side down, on the custard. Spread the glaze over the top of the cake. Refrigerate until chilled before cutting.

Per serving

CALORIES: 240 FAT: 14g PROTEIN: 3g CARBOHYDRATES: 29g SODIUM: 38mg CHOLESTEROL: 68mg FIBER: 1g

■ ■ ■

Rhubarb Meringue Dessert

I have fond memories of this dessert; a friend served something similar at my baby shower many years ago. I liked it so much that I developed my own version. Similar to a meringue pie, this dessert is great in the spring, when fresh rhubarb is plentiful.

MAKES 8 SERVINGS

CRUST

¼ cup finely chopped pecans

¾ cup flour blend (page 11)

2 tablespoons sugar

¼ teaspoon xanthan gum

¼ cup melted margarine (see note, page 23)

FILLING

3 large egg yolks

3 tablespoons sweet rice flour

1 cup sugar

3 cups finely diced rhubarb

1 teaspoon vanilla extract

1 drop red food coloring (optional)

MERINGUE

3 large egg whites

¼ teaspoon cream of tartar

¼ cup sugar

1. Preheat the oven to 325°F. Grease an 11 x 7-inch baking pan.

2. To make the crust: Process the pecans in a food processor until very fine. Add the flour blend, sugar, xanthan gum, and margarine and process until thoroughly blended. Pat into the prepared pan. Bake for 8 minutes, or until lightly browned. Set aside. Increase the oven temperature to 425°F.

3. To make the filling: In a heavy, nonreactive saucepan, combine the egg yolks, rice flour, sugar, and rhubarb. Cook over medium heat, stirring, for about 5 minutes, or until the mixture thickens. Stir in the vanilla and red food coloring, if using. Pour the filling over the crust.

4. To make the meringue: Beat the egg whites and cream of tartar until soft peaks form. Gradually beat in the sugar and beat until stiff peaks form. Spread the meringue over the rhubarb filling.

5. Bake until the meringue is light golden brown. (Browning time varies with different ovens; watch carefully so it doesn't burn.) Cool on a wire rack. Cut into 8 squares.

Per serving
CALORIES: 325 FAT: 9g PROTEIN: 4g CARBOHYDRATES: 60g SODIUM: 882mg CHOLESTEROL: 68mg FIBER: 1g

■ ■ ■

Crumb Crust for Pies

This crust is great for cheesecakes and no-bake pie fillings such as puddings and custards.

MAKES 1 (9-INCH) PIECRUST; 6 SERVINGS

1 cup crushed cookie crumbs [Vanilla Wafers (page 182), Chocolate Wafer Cookies (page 176), or Pamela's or Enjoy Life cookies]
4 tablespoons margarine (see note, page 23), at room temperature
1/4 cup finely chopped nuts or crushed cookie crumbs
2 tablespoons sugar

1. Combine all the ingredients in a food processor. Press into a 9-inch microwave-safe pie plate.
2. Cook for 2 to 3 minutes on High, until firm. Fill the crust with filling of your choice.

Per ⅙ of crust
CALORIES: 305 FAT: 19g PROTEIN: 3g CARBOHYDRATES: 34g SODIUM: 210mg CHOLESTEROL: 0mg FIBER: 0.5g

■ ■ ■

Piecrust of Dried Fruit & Nuts

Use this crust for puddings or fresh fruit pie fillings. It's crunchy and slightly tart and adds a very interesting note to smooth-textured fillings. You may vary the nuts as you wish.

MAKES 1 (9-INCH) PIECRUST; 6 SERVINGS

1 cup finely chopped dried apricots
1 cup finely ground pecans
1 tablespoon canola oil

1. Preheat the oven to 325°F. Grease a 9-inch pie plate. Combine the apricots, nuts, and oil in a food processor and process until well mixed. Press onto the bottom of the prepared pie plate.
2. Bake for 5 minutes. Fill the crust with filling of your choice.

Per ⅙ of crust
CALORIES: 150 FAT: 9g PROTEIN: 2g CARBOHYDRATES: 18g SODIUM: 3mg CHOLESTEROL: 0mg FIBER: 0.5g

■ ■ ■

✳ *Spiced Peach Pie*

*P*ie is the all-American dessert; this easy recipe allows you to indulge often. It works best with stone-fruit fillings like cherry, peach, or apricot. If you use your favorite fruit filling for a 9-inch pie, limit the amount of juice to 2 tablespoons.

MAKES 1 (9-INCH) DOUBLE-CRUST PIE;
8 SERVINGS

DOUBLE PIECRUST

1 cup Sorghum–Corn Flour Blend
   (page 11)
¾ cup tapioca flour
½ cup sweet rice flour
1 teaspoon guar gum
1 teaspoon xanthan gum
½ teaspoon salt
1 tablespoon sugar
½ cup shortening (see note, page 207)
2 tablespoons butter or margarine, softened
   (see note, page 23)
¼ cup milk (cow, rice, or soy)

SPICED PEACH FILLING

4 cups peeled, pitted, and sliced fresh peaches
   (about 6 medium)
½ cup sugar
¼ cup potato starch
2 teaspoons fresh lemon juice
½ teaspoon ground cinnamon

¼ teaspoon ground ginger
¼ teaspoon ground cardamom
¼ teaspoon salt

ASSEMBLY

1 egg beaten with 1 tablespoon water, for wash
1 teaspoon sugar

1. To make the crust: Combine the flour blend, tapioca flour, gums, salt, sugar, shortening, and butter in a food processor. Process until the mixture resembles coarse meal. Add the milk and process until the dough forms a ball. Flatten the dough to a 1-inch-thick disk, wrap tightly, and refrigerate for 1 hour so the liquids are well distributed throughout the dough.

2. To make the filling: Combine all the ingredients in a medium bowl. Let stand while rolling out the dough.

3. Massage the dough between your hands until it is warm and pliable, making it easier to handle. Divide into 2 equal pieces. Roll half of the dough into a 10-inch circle between 2 pieces of heavy-duty plastic wrap dusted with rice flour. (Use a damp paper towel between the countertop and plastic wrap to anchor the plastic wrap.) Move the rolling pin from the center of the dough to the outer edge, moving around the circle in clockwise fashion to assure uniform thickness. Keep remaining half wrapped tightly to avoid drying out.

4. Remove the top piece of plastic wrap and invert crust, centering it over a 9-inch nonstick pie plate. Remove the remaining

plastic wrap and press the dough into the plate. If the dough is hard to handle, press the entire bottom crust in place with your fingers.

5. Discard all but 2 tablespoons of the liquid in the filling mixture. Spoon the filling into the crust.

6. Preheat the oven to 375°F. Roll the remaining dough into a 10-inch circle between 2 pieces of plastic wrap. Invert and center on the filled crust. Don't remove the top piece of plastic wrap until the dough is centered. Shape a decorative edge around the rim of the pie plate. Freeze for 15 minutes.

7. Brush the top crust with the egg wash. Sprinkle with the sugar. Prick the crust several times with a fork so the steam can escape. Place on a nonstick baking sheet. Bake the pie on the lowest oven rack for 15 minutes to brown the bottom crust. Move to next higher oven rack and bake for 25 to 35 minutes, or until the crust is nicely browned. Cover loosely with foil if the edges brown too quickly. Cool completely on a wire rack before cutting.

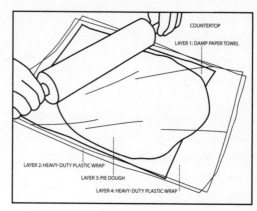

Piecrust

Per serving
CALORIES: 425 FAT: 17g PROTEIN: 3g CARBOHYDRATES: 72mg SODIUM: 235mg CHOLESTEROL: 23mg FIBER: 2g

Baked Single Crust

Following the instructions in steps 4 and 5, roll out half of the dough into a 10-inch circle and use to line a 9-inch nonstick pie plate. (Wrap and freeze remaining dough for later use.) Shape a dec-

orative ridge around the rim of pie plate. Prick the crust several times with a fork so it will lay flat during baking. Freeze the crust for 15 minutes.

Preheat the oven to 375°F. Place the pie plate on a baking sheet. Bake the crust on the lowest oven rack for 10 minutes. Move to the next highest oven rack and bake for 10 minutes, or until the crust rim is lightly browned. Cool on a rack before filling.

Per ⅛ of crust
CALORIES: 170 FAT: 8g PROTEIN: 1g CARBOHYDRATES: 24mg SODIUM: 85mg CHOLESTEROL: 15mg FIBER: 0.5g

■ ■ ■

Chocolate Soufflé

This is a very elegant, very special dessert. Put the prepared soufflés in the oven when you sit down to dinner. They'll be ready to eat when you're ready for dessert. Serve plain or with White Chocolate Topping (page 197).

MAKES 2 SERVINGS

¼ cup whipping cream or 3 tablespoons milk
   (cow, rice, or soy)
4 ounces bittersweet gluten-free, dairy-free
   chocolate
2 large egg yolks
1 teaspoon orange extract
1 teaspoon grated orange zest
3 tablespoons sugar
3 large egg whites
⅛ teaspoon cream of tartar

1. Heat the cream and chocolate in a heavy saucepan over low heat, stirring frequently, until the chocolate melts. Remove from the heat. With an electric mixer on medium speed, beat in the egg yolks, one yolk at a time. Stir in the orange extract and orange zest. Refrigerate for 5 minutes to cool.

2. Preheat oven to 375°F. Grease 1 (4-cup) or 2 (1¾-cup) soufflé dishes and dust with 1 tablespoon of the sugar.

3. With an electric mixer on high speed and clean beaters, beat the egg whites and cream of tartar in a medium bowl until soft peaks form. Gradually beat in the remaining 2 tablespoons sugar. Fold ¼ cup of the egg whites into the chocolate mixture, then gently fold in the remaining egg whites. Spoon the mixture into the prepared dish.

4. Bake the large soufflé for 30 minutes or the smaller soufflés for 20 minutes, or until soufflé rises but the center remains slightly soft. Serve immediately

---

Per serving

CALORIES: 550 FAT: 33g PROTEIN: 11g CARBOHYDRATES: 59g SODIUM: 107mg CHOLESTEROL: 251mg FIBER: 3g

■ ■ ■

Mexican Flan

This is an easy, almost foolproof version to make in the microwave oven. It is a creamy, tongue-soothing finale to a spicy Southwestern meal. The caramel sauce is exquisite. This recipe is dairy-based.

MAKES 6 SERVINGS

½ cup sugar
2 tablespoons water
4 large eggs
1 (14-ounce) can sweetened condensed milk
1 (12-ounce) can evaporated skim milk
½ cup half-and-half
2 teaspoons vanilla extract

1. Coat 6 (6-ounce) custard cups with cooking spray. Set aside.

2. In a 2-cup glass (not plastic) measuring cup, microwave the sugar and water on High for 5 to 7 minutes, or until the mixture boils

and turns a walnut-brown color. (Watch carefully after 5 minutes of cooking, since microwaves vary in power and the sugar can easily burn.) Quickly, pour the hot syrup evenly into the prepared custard cups.

3. In a large bowl, whisk the eggs until well blended; whisk in the remaining ingredients. Pour an equal amount into each custard cup. Arrange the custard cups in a circle in a microwave oven.

4. Microwave on Medium for 12 to 18 minutes, rotating the cups a quarter turn every 4 minutes. The flan is done when a knife inserted into the edges comes out clean but comes out thickly coated with custard when inserted in the centers. (The centers will firm up after chilling.)

5. Cool the flans on a wire rack for 30 minutes. Refrigerate for at least 4 to 6 hours before unmolding.

6. To unmold, run a thin knife around the edges of each flan and unmold onto a serving dish or into a bowl.

Per serving
CALORIES: 390 FAT: 11g PROTEIN: 14g CARBOHYDRATES: 61g SODIUM: 190mg CHOLESTEROL: 152mg FIBER: 0g

■ ■ ■

Natillas

This is a Mexican vanilla pudding that is light and refreshing. If, like me, you are concerned about eating uncooked eggs, see the note below.

MAKES 4 SERVINGS

2 large eggs, separated (see notes, below)
2 heaping tablespoons tapioca flour
2 cups whole milk (cow, rice, or soy)
¼ cup sugar
⅛ teaspoon salt
½ teaspoon vanilla extract
½ teaspoon ground cinnamon

1. In a medium bowl, beat the egg yolks and flour with an electric mixer on low speed to a smooth paste, about 1 minute. Beat in ½ cup of the milk; set aside.

2. In a medium, heavy saucepan, heat the sugar, remaining 1½ cups milk, and salt over medium heat, 1 to 3 minutes, or until bubbles form around the edge of the milk.

3. Reduce the heat to medium-low and, stirring constantly, slowly pour in the egg yolk–milk mixture in a steady stream. Cook, stirring, for 5 to 8 minutes, until the mixture thickens and leaves a path on the back of a spoon when your finger is drawn across it. Remove from the heat; stir in the vanilla.

Refrigerate the custard for 1 hour or place in the freezer for 15 minutes, then transfer it to the refrigerator until chilled.

4. With an electric mixer at high speed and clean beaters, beat the egg whites in a medium bowl until soft peaks form. Fold the egg whites into the custard. Transfer to a serving bowl. Sprinkle with the cinnamon.

Per serving

CALORIES: 175 FAT: 7g PROTEIN: 8g CARBOHYDRATES: 22g SODIUM: 158mg CHOLESTEROL: 123mg FIBER: 0.5g

Notes: Uncooked eggs should not be eaten by young children, the elderly, or anyone with a compromised immune system, because they may contain salmonella bacteria that can cause serious illness. Pasteurized eggs are available in many markets and are safe to eat raw in sauces or desserts that are not cooked.

Instead of raw egg whites, use dried egg whites or instant meringue mix, following the package directions. Instant meringue mix is in the baking section of grocery stores.

■ ■ ■

Bread Pudding with Lemon Sauce

This is a great way to use up leftover gluten-free Popovers (page 44) and French Bread (page 25). To reduce calories, use your favorite milk in place of the half-and-half.

MAKES 6 SERVINGS

BREAD PUDDING

2 cups milk (cow, rice, or soy)

½ cup sugar

4 large eggs

1 teaspoon grated lemon zest

1 teaspoon vanilla extract

1 teaspoon lemon extract

6 cups 1-inch cubes gluten-free bread

1 cup blueberries

LEMON SAUCE

1 cup half-and-half or ¾ cup milk (cow, rice, or soy)

3 large egg yolks

2 tablespoons sugar

1 teaspoon cornstarch

¼ cup honey

1 teaspoon lemon extract

1 teaspoon rum extract (optional)

1. Grease an 8-inch-square baking dish.

2. To make the pudding: Whisk together the milk, sugar, eggs, lemon zest, and vanilla, and lemon extract in a medium bowl.

3. Place half of the bread on the bottom of the prepared dish. Top with the blueberries and half of the egg mixture. Top with the remaining bread, then the remaining egg mixture. Let stand for 15 minutes, occasionally pressing down on bread.

4. Preheat the oven to 325°F. Bake the pudding for 45 minutes to 1 hour, or until the

top begins to brown. Cool the pudding for 10 to 15 minutes before serving.

5. To make the sauce: Bring the half-and-half to a simmer in a heavy pan. Whisk the egg yolks, sugar, and cornstarch in a medium bowl. Gradually whisk in the hot half-and-half. Return the mixture to the pan and cook, stirring, over medium-low heat for about 3 minutes or until the mixture thickens and leaves a path on the back of a spoon when your finger is drawn across it. Do not boil. Mix in the remaining ingredients. Spoon over the warm pudding.

Per serving
CALORIES: 640 FAT: 14g PROTEIN: 19g CARBOHYDRATES: 108g SODIUM: 913mg CHOLESTEROL: 170mg FIBER: 5g

■ ■ ■

Butterscotch Pudding

*E*xtremely rich and satisfying, this is a great dessert for company because you can make it ahead of time, and there's no last-minute preparation.

MAKES 4 SERVINGS

½ cup packed dark brown sugar
2 tablespoons cornstarch
¼ teaspoon salt
1½ cups evaporated skim milk or 1⅓ cups non-dairy milk [cow, rice (see note below), or soy]
1 large egg yolk

1 tablespoon butter or margarine (see note, page 23)
1 teaspoon vanilla extract
½ teaspoon butter-flavored extract (optional)
Whipped cream or shaved chocolate, for serving (optional)

1. In a large, heavy saucepan over medium heat, whisk the brown sugar, cornstarch, and salt. Gradually whisk in the milk. Whisk in the egg yolk and bring the mixture to a boil, whisking constantly. Immediately reduce the heat to low and boil for 1 minute. (This boiling time is critical because it develops the butterscotch flavor, but be careful; the mixture may splatter as it boils.)

2. Remove from the heat and stir in the butter, vanilla, and butter extract, if using. Divide equally among 4 dessert cups, cover, and refrigerate for 2 hours. Serve with a dollop of whipped cream, if desired.

Per serving
CALORIES: 160 FAT: 4g PROTEIN: 8g CARBOHYDRATES: 23g SODIUM: 273mg CHOLESTEROL: 64mg FIBER: 0g

*N*ote: If using rice milk, increase the cornstarch to 3 tablespoons.

■ ■ ■

Chocolate Pudding

This is a favorite "standby" dessert at our house. It can be prepared ahead of time and has a rich chocolate flavor. You can layer it with whipped cream, your favorite yogurt, or crushed gluten-free cookies. It can be a simple comfort food or fancy when layered in a pretty goblet.

MAKES 4 SERVINGS

⅓ cup granulated sugar or packed
    light brown sugar
2 tablespoons cornstarch
2 tablespoons unsweetened cocoa powder
1 teaspoon gluten-free instant espresso
    granules (optional)
⅛ teaspoon salt
1¾ cups skim milk [cow, rice (see note, page
    191), soy, or nut]
1 ounce gluten-free, dairy-free bittersweet
    chocolate
1 teaspoon vanilla extract

1. In a large, heavy saucepan over medium heat, whisk the sugar, cornstarch, cocoa powder, espresso granules, if using, and salt. Gradually whisk in the milk. Bring to a boil over medium heat, whisking constantly. Add the chocolate and cook, stirring constantly, for 1 minute.

2. Remove from the heat and stir in the vanilla. Pour into a bowl or 4 individual serving bowls. Cover and refrigerate for 2 hours.

Per serving
CALORIES: 165 FAT: 3g PROTEIN: 5g CARBOHYDRATES: 33g SODIUM: 134mg CHOLESTEROL: 2mg FIBER: 1.5g

■ ■ ■

Lemon Pudding

This smooth lemon pudding is great by itself. It also makes a great lemon meringue pie filling or layer it with whipped cream or lemon yogurt for a delightful parfait.

MAKES 6 SERVINGS

¾ cup sugar
1 tablespoon cornstarch
½ teaspoon grated lemon zest
⅓ cup water
⅓ cup fresh lemon juice
1 large egg
1 large egg yolk
1 tablespoon butter or margarine
    (see note, page 23)

1. Mix the sugar, cornstarch, and lemon zest in a heavy saucepan. Whisk in the water and lemon juice until blended. Bring to a boil over medium heat and boil, stirring constantly, for 1 minute. Remove from the heat.

2. Slightly beat the egg and egg yolk in a small bowl. Whisk 3 tablespoons of the hot lemon mixture into the egg mixture. Stirring constantly, add the egg mixture to the mixture in the pan. Cook over medium heat, stirring constantly, for 1 minute, or until thickened.

3. Remove from the heat. Stir in the butter. Pour into a serving bowl, cover loosely, and refrigerate until chilled.

Per serving
CALORIES: 145 FAT: 4g PROTEIN: 2g CARBOHYDRATES: 28g SODIUM: 32mg CHOLESTEROL: 76mg FIBER: 0.5g

▪ ▪ ▪

Vanilla Custard

This makes a rich, thick custard appropriate for Cream Puffs (below) or Vanilla Cream Pie (page 183). Or just eat it as vanilla pudding with a dollop of whipped cream or nondairy topping.

MAKES 4 SERVINGS; 1¼ CUPS

1 cup milk (cow, rice, or soy)
½ cup sugar
¼ cup cornstarch
4 large egg yolks, at room temperature
1 tablespoon butter or margarine
   (see note, page 23)
2 teaspoons vanilla extract

1. In a medium-heavy saucepan, heat the milk over medium heat just until hot.

2. In a small bowl, mix the sugar and cornstarch. In another medium bowl, beat the egg yolks with an electric mixer on medium speed until thick and lemon-colored. Slowly add the cornstarch mixture to the yolks, mixing thoroughly until smooth. With the electric mixer, gradually beat the hot milk into the yolk mixture.

3. Return the mixture to the same pan and cook over low heat, whisking constantly, for 2 minutes, or until the custard thickens.

4. Remove from the heat. Stir in the butter and vanilla. Transfer to a bowl, cover the surface of the custard with plastic wrap to prevent a skin from forming, and refrigerate until chilled. Stir before serving.

Per serving
CALORIES: 250 FAT: 10g PROTEIN: 6g CARBOHYDRATES: 34g SODIUM: 66mg CHOLESTEROL: 229mg FIBER: 0g

▪ ▪ ▪

Cream Puffs

Cream Puffs are one of the easiest and most foolproof desserts you can make with gluten-free flours. You can omit the whipped cream, and fill them with tuna or chicken salad for lunch.

MAKES 12 CREAM PUFFS; 6 SERVINGS

½ cup white rice flour

¼ cup potato starch

¾ cup water

5 tablespoons butter or margarine
  (see note, page 23)

2 teaspoons plus ¼ cup granulated sugar

¼ teaspoon salt

3 large eggs, at room temperature

½ cup whipping cream or nondairy topping

Powdered sugar, for garnish

1. Preheat the oven to 450°F. Grease a baking sheet or line with parchment paper. Set aside. Mix the rice flour and potato starch together in a small bowl and set aside.

2. Combine the water, butter, 2 teaspoons granulated sugar, and salt in a medium saucepan over medium-high heat and bring to a boil. As soon as the mixture comes to a boil, remove it from the heat and stir in the flour mixture, all at once. Return the mixture to the heat; cook, stirring with a wooden spoon and pressing the mixture against the side of the pan, until it pulls away from the side.

3. Remove the dough from the heat. Beat in the eggs, one at a time, beating with an electric mixer at Low speed after each addition until smooth before adding the next egg.

4. Drop mounds of the dough onto prepared baking sheet. Each mound should measure about 2 inches in diameter and 1½ to 2 inches in height. With a wet finger, smooth any points of dough that stick up, because these points will brown faster and may burn. (Use a spring-action, 2-inch ice cream scoop to make even, uniformly shaped cream puffs.)

5. Bake for 20 minutes, then reduce the oven temperature to 350°F and bake for 15 minutes longer, or until the cream puffs are deep golden brown. Remove from the oven and immediately cut a 1-inch horizontal slit in the side of each cream puff, where you'll eventually cut them completely in half. Cool on wire racks.

6. Whip the cream until soft peaks form. Gradually beat in the remaining ¼ cup granulated sugar until stiff peaks form. When the cream puffs are cool, cut them completely in half horizontally along the slit and fill with the whipped cream. Dust with powdered sugar.

Per serving
CALORIES: 260 FAT: 16g PROTEIN: 4g CARBOHYDRATES: 27g SODIUM: 218mg CHOLESTEROL: 129mg FIBER: <1g

VARIATION

Cream Puffs with Vanilla Custard Filling
Fill with Vanilla Custard (page 193) instead of whipped cream.

Per serving
CALORIES: 280 FAT: 15g PROTEIN: 6g CARBOHYDRATES: 31g SODIUM: 236mg CHOLESTEROL: 194mg FIBER: 0.5g

■ ■ ■

Crepes

Crepes have unlimited uses as "containers" for desserts or entrées. Try filling them with cream cheese and top with strawberries or blueberries. Or fold them in quarters, and dip in melted orange marmalade for an easy crepe Suzette.

MAKES ABOUT 12 CREPES; 6 SERVINGS

⅓ cup white rice flour

⅓ cup brown rice flour

½ teaspoon xanthan gum

½ teaspoon unflavored gelatin powder

⅛ teaspoon salt

¾ cup milk (cow, rice, or soy)

2 large eggs

2 teaspoons canola oil

1 teaspoon vanilla extract

1. Combine all the ingredients in a blender and process until smooth. If possible, refrigerate (in the blender jar) for about 30 minutes.

2. Heat an 8-inch skillet or seasoned crepe pan over medium-high heat until a drop of water dances on the surface. Spray the pan with cooking spray. Pour scant 2 tablespoons of the batter into the pan and immediately tilt the pan to coat the bottom evenly. Cook until the underside of the crepe is lightly browned; turn and cook the other side for about 20 to 30 seconds. (Often the first crepe will not turn out as well as succeeding ones because of the temperature of the pan. If so, discard the first crepe.) Repeat with the remaining batter.

Per serving

CALORIES: 140 FAT: 4g PROTEIN: 4g CARBOHYDRATES: 24g SODIUM: 79mg CHOLESTEROL: 61mg FIBER: 0.5g

■ ■ ■

Chocolate Glaze

Use this glaze on top of the Mexican Chocolate Cake (page 168) or on fresh fruit or puddings. Whole milk (or nondairy liquid) can be substituted for the half-and-half.

MAKES ABOUT 1½ CUPS; 10 SERVINGS

¼ cup half-and-half

3 ounces Mexican chocolate (Ibarra brand)

1 ounce bittersweet chocolate

2 tablespoons canola oil

1 tablespoon honey

1 tablespoon pure maple syrup

1. In a small, heavy saucepan, heat the half-and-half over medium heat for 5 minutes or until bubbles form around the edge of the half-and-half. Set aside.

2. In the top of a double boiler over simmering water (or in a microwave oven on Low setting), heat the chocolates, oil, honey, and

maple syrup, stirring frequently, for about 5 minutes, or until the chocolate melts.

3. Remove the chocolate mixture from the heat. Stir the half-and-half into the chocolate mixture. Cool before using.

Per 2 tablespoons
CALORIES: 100 FAT: 7g PROTEIN: 1g CARBOHYDRATES: 10g SODIUM: 4mg CHOLESTEROL: 2mg FIBER: 0.5g

■ ■ ■

Seven-Minute Coffee Frosting

Don't let those elegant frostings with all the dips and swirls intimidate you. You can do it, and it is extremely easy. Use this delicious frosting for the Spice Cake (page 170). It's also wonderful on the Chocolate Cake (page 167). You can vary the flavor: omit the coffee for a vanilla frosting or use lemon or orange extract for a citrus flavor.

MAKES ENOUGH FROSTING FOR AN 8-INCH LAYER CAKE; 10 SERVINGS

1 teaspoon gluten-free instant coffee or
  espresso granules
1 teaspoon very hot water or hot brewed coffee
3 large egg whites
1¼ cups sugar
¼ teaspoon cream of tartar

3 tablespoons cold water
1 teaspoon vanilla extract

1. Dissolve the coffee in the hot water; set aside.

2. In a double boiler over boiling water, combine the egg whites, sugar, cream of tartar, and cold water. Beat with an electric mixer on high speed for about 7 minutes, or until soft peaks form.

3. Remove the meringue from the heat and stir in the vanilla and reserved coffee liquid with a spatula until desired spreading consistency. Use immediately.

Per serving
CALORIES: 105 FAT: 0.5g PROTEIN: 1g CARBOHYDRATES: 27g SODIUM: 21mg CHOLESTEROL: 0mg FIBER: 0g

■ ■ ■

Raspberry Sauce

This sauce is great on ice cream, as a coulis (pronounced cou-LEE) under desserts such as cakes or cheesecakes, or I sometimes use it as a filling for layer cakes. You can also baste Cornish game hens with it. For a larger amount, double or triple the ingredients.

MAKES ABOUT ¼ CUP

3 tablespoons raspberry jam (use all-fruit
  seedless type)

1 teaspoon orange extract

1 tablespoon orange juice

Combine all ingredients in small saucepan. Heat, stirring constantly, over medium heat until the jam has melted. Cool before using.

Per tablespoon

CALORIES: 50 FAT: 0g PROTEIN:1g CARBOHYDRATES: 10g SODIUM: 6mg CHOLESTEROL: 0mg FIBER: 0.5g

■ ■ ■

White Chocolate Topping

This topping can be used on the Chocolate Brownies (page 175) or Chocolate Soufflé (page 187). It's also good over fresh fruits.

MAKES ABOUT 1¼ CUPS; 4 SERVINGS

1 ounce gluten-free white chocolate

1 cup Yogurt Cheese (page 94) or soft, silken tofu

1 tablespoon sugar

¼ cup milk (cow, rice, or soy)

½ teaspoon grated orange zest

1 tablespoon fresh orange juice

1. Dice the chocolate into very small pieces.
2. Combine the remaining ingredients in a blender and blend until very smooth. Stir in the chocolate pieces. Serve immediately.

Per serving

CALORIES: 90 FAT: 5g PROTEIN: 3g CARBOHYDRATES: 11g SODIUM: 34mg CHOLESTEROL: 9mg FIBER: 0.5g

■ ■ ■

Hot Fudge Sauce

This delectable, rich sauce keeps in the refrigerator for up to one month. Just warm in the microwave before serving.

MAKES 3 CUPS; 12 SERVINGS

2 cups packed light brown sugar

⅔ cup unsweetened cocoa powder (not Dutch)

1 cup evaporated skim milk or soy or rice milk

2 tablespoons butter or margarine (see note, page 23)

1 teaspoon vanilla extract

½ teaspoon salt

In a heavy saucepan, mix the sugar and cocoa. Gradually stir in the milk. Bring to a boil over medium heat, stirring constantly. Boil, stirring constantly, for 1 minute. Reduce the heat to low and cook, beating with a spoon, until smooth. Remove from the heat and stir in the butter, vanilla, and salt.

Per ¼ cup

CALORIES: 145 FAT: 4g PROTEIN: 2g CARBOHYDRATES: 28g SODIUM: 141mg CHOLESTEROL: 11mg FIBER: 1.5g

10. Breakfast Dishes

Breakfast is perhaps the most important meal of the day. If you're like me, it's also your favorite meal. It helps wake us up and provides our bodies with the necessary nutrients and energy to start the day.

Unfortunately, many of the foods we eat at breakfast or brunch—toast, muffins, pancakes, doughnuts, and biscuits—are made with wheat. But you can make them all with the delicious recipes from this chapter.

When it comes to hot cereal, most gluten-free cooks think of rice as their only safe option, but there are many other choices. Nutrient-packed amaranth, buckwheat, and quinoa are great for breakfast, topped with sugar, cinnamon, honey, maple syrup, brown sugar, fresh fruit, jam, jelly, or nuts.

I especially miss those hearty "stick-to-your-ribs" hot cereals, so I have included a chart on cooking grains (see page 59) in the Grains & Beans chapter.

Biscuits and Gravy

Hot biscuits, fresh from the oven, are topped with creamy, soul-soothing gravy. I know this is typically a breakfast entrée; however, in some parts of the country folks add dried beef, and it becomes dinner.

MAKES 4 SERVINGS

Biscuits (page 206)
$\frac{1}{3}$ cup sweet rice flour
4 cups milk (cow, rice, or soy)
$\frac{1}{4}$ pound Country Sausage (page 158)
1 teaspoon salt
$\frac{1}{4}$ teaspoon dried thyme
$\frac{1}{2}$ teaspoon ground black pepper
$\frac{1}{4}$ cup chopped fresh parsley, for garnish

1. Have the biscuits baked and ready. Mix the flour with $\frac{1}{2}$ cup of the milk; set aside.

2. In a heavy saucepan, brown the sausage, stirring to break up the meat. With a slotted spoon, transfer the sausage to a plate and keep warm.

3. Stir the flour mixture, salt, thyme, pepper, and remaining $3\frac{1}{2}$ cups milk into the drippings remaining in the skillet. Cook, stirring constantly, over medium heat until the gravy thickens. Stir in the sausage.

4. Spoon the gravy over warm biscuits. Garnish with the parsley.

Per serving
CALORIES: 410 FAT: 23g PROTEIN: 14g CARBOHYDRATES: 37g SODIUM: 990mg CHOLESTEROL: 54mg FIBER: 0.5g

■ ■ ■

Quiche Lorraine

This quiche has an unusual crust: crispy potatoes. Nondairy cheeses do not work in this recipe.

MAKES 4 SERVINGS

3 cups grated, peeled potatoes
2 tablespoons canola oil
1 onion, diced
1 bacon slice, chopped
4 large eggs
1 cup whole milk (cow, rice, soy)
$\frac{1}{4}$ teaspoon salt
$\frac{1}{8}$ teaspoon ground white pepper
$\frac{1}{8}$ teaspoon ground nutmeg
1 tablespoon tapioca flour
$1\frac{1}{2}$ cups diced Swiss cheese
$\frac{1}{4}$ cup grated Parmesan cheese (cow or soy)

1. Preheat the oven to 425°F. Coat a 9-inch pie plate with cooking spray. Toss the potatoes and oil in a bowl and press evenly over the bottom and sides of the prepared pie plate. Bake for 30 minutes, or until lightly browned. Use foil to cover the edge if it

browns too quickly. Set aside. Reduce the oven temperature to 350°F.

2. Meanwhile, in a heavy skillet over medium heat, cook the onion and bacon, stirring constantly, until the bacon is crisp and the onion is lightly browned. Set aside.

3. In a bowl, combine the eggs, milk, salt, pepper, and nutmeg. Stir in the onion and bacon. Toss the flour with the Swiss cheese and add to the egg mixture.

4. Pour the egg mixture into the baked shell. Sprinkle the Parmesan cheese on top. Bake for 45 minutes, or until the center is set and a knife inserted in the center comes out clean. Serve immediately.

Per serving
CALORIES: 270 FAT: 18g PROTEIN: 19g CARBOHYDRATES: 12g SODIUM: 300mg CHOLESTEROL: 155mg FIBER: 0.5g

VARIATION

Substitute a 9-inch Baked Single Crust (page 187) for the potatoes and oil.

Per serving with pastry crust
CALORIES: 290 FAT: 23g PROTEIN: 19g CARBOHYDRATES: 9g SODIUM: 476mg CHOLESTEROL: 187mg FIBER: 0.5g

■ ■ ■

⋇Ham and Egg Breakfast Casserole

This dish makes a wonderful Sunday brunch, and because you make it the night before, you're free to do other things while it bakes. Use your leftover gluten-free Sandwich Bread (page 35) or French Bread (page 25). You may use your favorite nondairy Cheddar and Monterey Jack cheeses, if you wish.

MAKES 6 SERVINGS

12 slices gluten-free white bread, or enough to make 2 layers in pan

1 cup shredded Cheddar cheese

1 cup shredded Monterey Jack cheese

2 cups diced Canadian-style bacon

1 tablespoon finely chopped onion

¼ cup grated Parmesan cheese (cow or soy)

4 large eggs

2 cups milk (cow, rice, or soy)

1 teaspoon Lea & Perrins Worcestershire sauce

1 teaspoon dry mustard (see note, page 68)

2 tablespoons chopped fresh parsley

1. Grease a 13 x 9-inch nonstick pan. Cover the bottom of the prepared pan with half of the bread slices.

2. Sprinkle ½ cup *each* of the Cheddar and Monterey Jack cheeses over the bread. Sprin-

kle the bacon, onion, and Parmesan cheese on top. Make another layer of bread. Sprinkle with the remaining Cheddar and Jack cheeses.

3. In a large bowl, beat the eggs, milk, Worcestershire sauce, and mustard. Pour over the cheeses. Cover and refrigerate overnight.

4. Preheat the oven to 350°F. Bake for 45 to 60 minutes, or until the top browns. Sprinkle with the parsley before serving.

Per serving

CALORIES: 380 FAT: 19g PROTEIN: 26g CARBOHYDRATES: 24g SODIUM: 1,315mg CHOLESTEROL: 155mg FIBER: 1g

■ ■ ■

Huevos Rancheros

*U*se homemade Corn Tortillas (page 42) or purchased ones for this traditional Southwestern breakfast.

MAKES 6 SERVINGS

2 tablespoons canola oil

6 Corn Tortillas (page 42) or purchased
   gluten-free corn tortillas

½ cup chopped onion

1 garlic clove, minced

4 large tomatoes, seeded and diced

1 (4-ounce) can diced green chiles, drained

¼ teaspoon dried oregano

¼ teaspoon ground cumin

½ teaspoon salt, plus extra for eggs

⅛ teaspoon ground white pepper, plus
   extra for eggs

6 large eggs

1 cup shredded Monterey Jack cheese or
   nondairy cheese of your choice

½ cup chopped fresh cilantro

1. Preheat the oven to 250°F. Heat the oil in a small, heavy skillet over medium heat. Using tongs, dip each tortilla, one at a time, into the hot oil for 8 to 10 seconds, until limp.

2. Line a 10 x 6-inch baking dish with the tortillas, letting the edges of the tortillas extend a little up the sides of the dish. Cover with foil and keep warm in the oven.

3. In the same skillet (sprayed with cooking spray if needed), sauté the onion and garlic over medium-low heat for 5 to 8 minutes, until tender. Stir in the tomatoes, chiles, oregano, cumin, salt, and pepper. Simmer, uncovered, for 10 minutes. Spoon the mixture over the tortillas.

4. Wipe the skillet clean with paper towels and coat with cooking spray. Over medium heat, break the eggs into the skillet and sprinkle lightly with salt and pepper. When the whites are set and edges cooked, add 1 tablespoon water. Cover the skillet and cook the eggs to desired degree of doneness.

5. Place an oven rack in broil position and turn the temperature control to broil setting. Carefully place the cooked eggs over the sauce in the baking dish. Sprinkle with cheese. Place under the broiler for 1 to 2 minutes, or

until the cheese melts. Top with the cilantro. Serve at once.

Per serving
CALORIES: 254 FAT: 15g PROTEIN: 12g CARBOHYDRATES: 18g SODIUM: 430mg CHOLESTEROL: 197mg FIBER: 3g

Note: If you are fortunate enough to have fresh green New Mexico chiles, use 1 small green chile that has been roasted, peeled, seeded, and finely chopped. Remember, chiles can be hot; use them sparingly at first and wear gloves when handling.

■ ■ ■

Mexican Tortilla Casserole

This dish makes a wonderful Southwestern Sunday brunch dish. You may use nondairy cheeses for the Cheddar and Monterey Jack cheeses. You may substitute your favorite Mexican salsa for the canned tomatoes and herbs.

MAKES 4 SERVINGS

2 (14.5-ounce) cans Mexican-style tomatoes
½ teaspoon dried oregano
½ teaspoon dried sage
½ cup chopped fresh cilantro
1½ cups shredded Monterey Jack cheese
1½ cups shredded Cheddar cheese

10 Corn Tortillas (page 42) or use purchased gluten-free corn tortillas
½ cup diced cooked pork
½ cup sliced black olives
½ cup guacamole
¼ cup sour cream or sour cream alternative

1. Preheat the oven to 450°F. Spray 2 (8-inch) pie plates with cooking spray.

2. For the sauce, combine the tomatoes, oregano, sage, and cilantro in a food processor and purée until smooth. Mix the cheeses in a bowl.

3. Pour ¼ cup of the sauce into one of the prepared pie plates. Top with 1 tortilla, ⅓ cup of the cheese, and ¼ cup of the sauce. Repeat the layers 3 more times. Top with the fifth tortilla, ¼ cup pork, ¼ cup sauce, and 2 tablespoons of the cheese. Repeat with the remaining ingredients in the second pie plate.

4. Bake for 12 to 15 minutes, or until the cheese melts and the sauce is bubbly. Cut each casserole in half to serve. Garnish with the olives, guacamole, and sour cream.

Per serving
CALORIES: 625 FAT: 50g PROTEIN: 36g CARBOHYDRATES: 9g SODIUM: 860mg CHOLESTEROL: 139mg FIBER: 2g

VARIATION

Meatless Mexican Tortilla Casserole
Omit the pork.

Per serving
CALORIES: 450 FAT: 36g PROTEIN: 23g CARBOHYDRATES:
10g SODIUM: 697mg CHOLESTEROL: 88mg FIBER: 2g

■ ■ ■

Mexican Brunch Casserole

A mildly spicy dish, it can be assembled the night before. You may use nondairy Cheddar and Monterey Jack cheeses, if you wish.

MAKES 6 SERVINGS

2 cups ½-inch cubes French bread (page 25)
4 ounces Chorizo (page 157)
1 small onion, chopped
4 large eggs
1¼ cups milk (cow, rice, or soy)
1 teaspoon dry mustard (see note, page 68)
½ (4-ounce) can green chiles, drained
½ cup finely chopped fresh cilantro
¼ teaspoon salt
⅛ teaspoon ground black pepper
½ cup shredded Monterey Jack cheese
½ cup shredded smoked Cheddar cheese
1½ cups purchased gluten-free Mexican
   tomato-chile salsa
½ cup guacamole (optional)
½ cup gluten-free, light sour cream or sour
   cream alternative (optional)

1. Preheat the oven 325°F. Place the bread on a baking sheet and bake for 10 to 15 minutes, or until lightly toasted. (This is optional, but adds a richer flavor.)

2. Cook the sausage and onion in a large, heavy skillet over medium heat, stirring to break up the meat, until the sausage is cooked and the onion is lightly browned. Drain.

3. Beat the eggs, milk, mustard, chiles, cilantro, salt, and pepper in a large bowl until thoroughly blended.

4. Grease an 8-inch-square baking dish. Place the bread in the bottom of the prepared dish. Spoon the sausage and onion mixture over the bread. Sprinkle with the cheeses. Pour the egg mixture over the top. Cover and refrigerate overnight.

5. Preheat the oven to 350°F. Uncover the dish and bake for 40 to 45 minutes, or until the casserole is set and bubbling. Serve with the salsa. Top with the guacamole and/or sour cream, if desired.

Per serving
CALORIES: 550 FAT: 26g PROTEIN: 24g CARBOHYDRATES:
50g SODIUM: 1,239mg CHOLESTEROL: 193mg FIBER: 4g

■ ■ ■

Stuffed French Toast

This is a classic at our house for Sunday brunch, and it always gets many compliments. You can vary the stuffing, perhaps adding a thin slice of proscuitto along with the cream cheese.

MAKES 10 PIECES

8 ounces cream cheese, softened, or firm silken
   tofu, creamed
1½ teaspoons vanilla extract
½ teaspoon orange extract or grated
   orange zest
½ cup chopped walnuts
1 loaf French Bread (page 25)
4 large eggs
1 cup whole milk (cow, rice, or soy)
½ teaspoon ground nutmeg
1½ cups apricot preserves
½ cup orange juice

1. Preheat the oven to 250°F. Beat the cream cheese, 1 teaspoon of the vanilla, and the orange extract until fluffy. Stir in the nuts.

2. Cut the bread into 10 slices, each 1½ inches thick. Cut a pocket in the top crust of each slice by slicing halfway through the crust. Fill the pocket of each slice with 1½ tablespoons of the cream cheese mixture.

3. In a medium bowl, beat the eggs, milk, remaining ½ teaspoon vanilla, and nutmeg. Using tongs, dip both sides of each bread slice in the egg mixture. Heat a lightly oiled griddle over medium-low heat. Cook the bread, in batches, on both sides until lightly browned. Transfer the toast as it is done to a baking sheet and keep warm in the oven until all the bread slices are cooked.

4. Meanwhile, heat the apricot preserves and orange juice in a microwave-safe bowl in the microwave until the preserves have melted. To serve, drizzle the apricot mixture over the French toast. (For added flavor, drizzle some apricot mixture over the bread slices while they warm in the oven. Pass the extra apricot mixture at serving time.)

Per serving
CALORIES: 315 FAT: 9g PROTEIN: 10g CARBOHYDRATES: 50g SODIUM: 390mg CHOLESTEROL: 88mg FIBER: 2g

VARIATION

Stuffed Raisin-Bread French Toast
Use Raisin Bread (page 32) instead of the French Bread.

Per piece
CALORIES: 365 FAT: 12g PROTEIN: 11g CARBOHYDRATES: 55g SODIUM: 317mg CHOLESTEROL: 119mg FIBER: 2g

■ ■ ■

Eggs Benedict

*U*se your own homemade English Muffins in this dish. It features Canadian-style bacon (lower in fat than ham) and low-fat Hollandaise Sauce (page 84).

MAKES 4 SERVINGS

1⅓ cups Hollandaise Sauce (page 84)

4 English Muffins (page 22)

8 slices Canadian-style bacon

8 large eggs

¼ cup chopped fresh parsley

Sweet paprika, for garnish

1. Make the Hollandaise Sauce and keep warm in a double boiler over warm water. Cut the muffins in half and warm in the microwave or wrap in foil and warm in a 250°F oven.

2. Meanwhile, warm the bacon in the microwave to serving temperature. Poach the eggs to desired doneness.

3. Arrange 2 halves of a muffin on each of 4 plates. Top each half with a bacon slice and a poached egg. Top with the sauce. Sprinkle with the parsley and paprika.

Per serving

CALORIES: 435 FAT: 20g PROTEIN: 29g CARBOHYDRATES: 33g SODIUM: 1,719mg CHOLESTEROL: 407mg FIBER: 0.5g

▪ ▪ ▪

Granola

Commercial prepared granolas can be very high in fat and sugar, and they often contain wheat flakes or wheat germ. By making your own, you can control the sugar and fat *and* you're sure there's no wheat!

MAKES 12 (½-CUP) SERVINGS

5 cups rolled rice flakes (see note, page 206) or puffed rice or corn

1 teaspoon ground cinnamon

½ cup shelled sunflower seeds

½ cup slivered almonds

½ cup unsweetened coconut flakes

2 teaspoons vanilla extract

2 teaspoons canola oil

½ cup light corn syrup

½ cup golden raisins

Preheat the oven to 300°F. Spray a baking sheet with cooking spray. Combine all the ingredients, except the raisins, in a medium bowl. Spread on the prepared baking sheet. Bake for 30 to 40 minutes, stirring every 10 minutes to ensure even browning, until lightly browned. Stir in the raisins. Cool and store in an airtight container for up to 1 week.

Per serving

CALORIES: 400 FAT: 12g PROTEIN: 14g CARBOHYDRATES: 62g SODIUM: 27mg CHOLESTEROL: 0mg FIBER: 1g

VARIATION

Trail Mix

Add dried fruit, such as apricots or cranberries, or the candy of your choice to the cooled granola, and you have a tasty trail mix.

Note: Rolled rice flakes are available at health food stores or at www.vitamincottage.com or www.enjoylifefoods.com.

■ ■ ■

Biscuits

Biscuits are the all-American food and so versatile: eat them with jam or jelly for breakfast or as Biscuits and Gravy (page 199). For a dinner entrée, top them with creamed chicken. For the best results have all the ingredients at room temperature. If you want to transform the biscuits into shortbread, add more sugar to the recipe (see variation, below).

MAKES 12 BISCUITS

1 cup flour blend (page 11)

½ cup cornstarch or potato starch

1 tablespoon sugar

2 teaspoons baking powder

1 teaspoon xanthan gum

1 teaspoon guar gum

½ teaspoon salt

¼ teaspoon baking soda

¼ cup shortening (see note, below)

½ cup milk (cow, rice, or soy)

1 large egg white

White rice flour, for dusting dough

1. Preheat the oven to 350°F. Grease a large baking sheet or line with parchment paper.

2. Combine the flour blend, cornstarch, sugar, baking powder, xanthan gum, guar gum, salt, baking soda, and shortening in a food processor and pulse until the mixture has the texture of large bread crumbs.

3. Add the milk and egg white and process until the mixture forms a ball. If a ball doesn't form, add water, 1 tablespoon at a time, and process until it does. The dough will be somewhat soft.

4. Place the dough on the prepared baking sheet. Lightly dust the dough with white rice flour. Gently pat to ¾-inch thickness. Cut into 2-inch circles with a biscuit cutter. Reshape trimmings and pat into ¾-inch thickness; cut more circles. If dough is sticky, lightly dust with more rice flour. Arrange circles about 1 inch apart on baking sheet.

5. Bake for 10 to 15 minutes, until lightly browned. Transfer to a wire rack to cool slightly. Serve warm.

Per biscuit
CALORIES: 145 FAT: 5g PROTEIN: 1g CARBOHYDRATES: 25g SODIUM: 185mg CHOLESTEROL: 4mg FIBER: .05g

VARIATION

Shortbread
Increase the sugar to ⅓ cup sugar. Cut into 12 pieces and bake as directed.

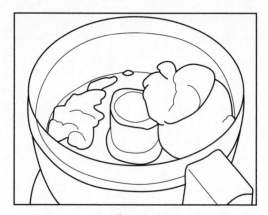

Biscuits

Per piece
CALORIES: 165 FAT: 5g PROTEIN: 1g CARBOHYDRATES: 31g CHOLESTEROL: 4mg SODIUM: 185mg FIBER: .05g

Note: Nonhydrogenated, trans fat–free shortenings by Spectrum or Smart Balance or Earth Balance are available at health food stores.

■ ■ ■

Pancakes

*A*merica's favorite breakfast is as easy as 1-2-3! See the variation below for make-ahead directions.

MAKES ABOUT 8 PANCAKES; 4 SERVINGS

2 large eggs
⅓ **cup milk (cow, rice, soy, or nut)**

½ **cup flour blend (page 11)**
1 teaspoon baking powder
½ **teaspoon baking soda**
1 teaspoon sugar
¼ **teaspoon salt**
1 teaspoon vanilla extract
1 tablespoon canola oil, plus oil for frying

1. Blend the eggs and milk in a blender or whisk in a medium bowl. Add the remaining ingredients and blend thoroughly.

2. Lightly oil a large nonstick skillet and heat over medium heat. Pour ¼ cup batter into skillet and cook 3 to 5 minutes, until tops are bubbly. Turn and cook for 2 to 3 minutes, until golden brown.

Each serving
CALORIES: 190 FAT: 7g PROTEIN: 5g CARBOHYDRATES: 29g SODIUM: 434mg CHOLESTEROL: 94mg FIBER: 0.5g

VARIATION

Make-Ahead Pancake Mix
Double or triple the amount of the dry ingredients (flour, baking powder, baking soda, sugar, and salt) and store in your pantry in an airtight container. For each batch of pancakes, combine ½ cup plus 1 tablespoon of the mix with 2 eggs, ⅓ cup milk, 1 teaspoon vanilla, and 1 tablespoon oil.

■ ■ ■

German Puffed Pancakes

This pancake puffs up as it bakes, creating lots of little indentations for the toppings. This was my son's favorite breakfast when he was a little boy. I still fix it for him now even though he is a grown man and has a son of his own.

MAKES 4 SERVINGS

3 large eggs
¼ cup flour blend (page 11)
¼ teaspoon salt
⅓ cup milk (cow, rice, or soy)
1 tablespoon butter or margarine (see note, page 23), at room temperature
Toppings (below)

1. Preheat the oven to 450°F. Grease a 9- or 10-inch cast-iron or other ovenproof skillet or 2 small (about 4-inch) ovenproof dishes.

2. In a blender, beat the eggs until thick and fluffy. Gradually add the flour blend, salt, and milk and blend until well mixed. Beat in the butter.

3. Pour the batter into the prepared skillet. Bake for 10 to 15 minutes for 9- or 10-inch pan (8 to 12 minutes for 4-inch pan), or until puffed and lightly browned. After removing from the oven, the center will fall slightly, making an indentation for a topping. Imme-

diately, spoon one of the following toppings over the pancake.

Each serving (without topping)
CALORIES: 120 FAT: 6g PROTEIN: 5g CARBOHYDRATES: 11g SODIUM: 213mg CHOLESTEROL: 144mg FIBER: 0.5g

TOPPINGS

Apple Topping

Peel, core, and slice 2 Granny Smith apples. Toss with 1 teaspoon cinnamon and ¼ cup sugar. Microwave on High for 5 to 7 minutes, or until the apples are tender. Spoon apples on top of baked pancake and dust with powdered sugar. Serve warm.

Each pancake with Apple Topping
CALORIES: 200 FAT: 6g PROTEIN: 5g CARBOHYDRATES: 31g SODIUM: 214mg CHOLESTEROL: 144mg FIBER: 1.5g

Eggs and Bacon Topping

Top each serving of pancakes with 1 scrambled egg and crumbled bacon strip. Sprinkle with chopped parsley. Serve immediately.

Each pancake with Egg and Bacon Topping
CALORIES: 215 FAT: 14g PROTEIN: 12g CARBOHYDRATES: 11g SODIUM: 368mg CHOLESTEROL: 330mg FIBER: 0.5g

■ ■ ■

Waffles

Waffles are a special treat for breakfast. Make a whole batch, then freeze any leftovers for another morning. They reheat nicely in the toaster, or they can be warmed gently in a 325°F oven until they reach serving temperature. The dimensions and number of waffles yielded by this recipe will vary, depending on your waffle maker.

MAKES 4 (8-INCH) WAFFLES; 8 SERVINGS

1 ¾ cups flour blend (page 11)

1 tablespoon sugar or honey

2 teaspoons baking powder

1 teaspoon salt

2 large eggs

¼ cup canola oil

1 ¼ cups buttermilk or 1 ½ tablespoons cider
  vinegar plus enough milk (cow, rice, or soy)
  to make 1 ¼ cups

1 teaspoon vanilla extract

1. Heat a waffle iron and coat with cooking spray. Sift the flour blend, sugar, baking powder, and salt into a small bowl. Beat eggs well in a large bowl. Add the oil, buttermilk, vanilla extract, and sifted dry ingredients; beat just until blended.

2. Pour one-fourth of the batter onto a preheated waffle iron or use the amount spec-ified by the manufacturer. Close and bake for 4 to 6 minutes, until the steaming stops. Repeat with remaining batter.

Per serving

CALORIES: 280 FAT: 9g PROTEIN: 4g CARBOHYDRATES: 48g SODIUM: 411mg CHOLESTEROL: 47mg FIBER: 0.5g

■ ■ ■

Corn Waffles

These waffles are great for breakfast topped with pepper jelly, or serve them with a cream sauce containing fish, meat, or chicken for a dinner entrée. The cornmeal lends an interesting twist to this old favorite.

MAKES 4 (8-INCH) WAFFLES

1 cup yellow cornmeal

1 cup flour blend (page 11)

1 tablespoon baking powder

1 teaspoon xanthan gum

¼ teaspoon salt

3 large eggs

1 (8-ounce) carton plain yogurt or ⅔ cup
  nondairy milk

½ cup milk (cow, rice, or soy)

¼ cup canola oil

Maple syrup or honey, to serve

1. In a large mixing bowl, stir the cornmeal, flour blend, baking powder, xanthan gum, and salt.

2. In a separate bowl, whisk the eggs, yogurt, milk, and oil until well blended. Add the egg mixture to the dry ingredients all at once. Stir just until combined but still lumpy.

3. Preheat a waffle iron. Pour about one-fourth of the batter onto the hot waffle iron. Follow the manufacturer's directions for cooking. Repeat with the remaining batter. Serve warm with maple syrup.

Per waffle
CALORIES: 215 FAT: 10g PROTEIN: 6g CARBOHYDRATES: 27g SODIUM: 250mg CHOLESTEROL: 70mg FIBER: 2g

VARIATION

Blue Corn Waffles
Substitute ½ cup blue cornmeal for ½ cup of the yellow cornmeal.

■ ■ ■

Baked Doughnuts

*E*verybody likes doughnuts, but most of us don't need that much fat in our diets. These doughnuts are baked rather than fried, but without any loss of flavor.

MAKES 12 DOUGHNUTS

DOUGHNUTS

2 cups flour blend (page 11)

2 teaspoons xanthan gum

1 teaspoon unflavored gelatin powder

1½ teaspoons baking powder

1½ teaspoons baking soda

½ teaspoon salt

2 teaspoons ground cinnamon

¼ teaspoon ground cloves

¼ teaspoon ground nutmeg

¼ teaspoon ground allspice

1 large egg, lightly beaten

⅔ cup packed dark brown sugar

½ cup apple juice frozen concentrate, thawed

⅓ cup pure maple syrup

⅓ cup strained applesauce or prune baby food

⅓ cup plain yogurt or ¼ cup milk (cow, rice, or soy)

¼ cup canola oil

FROSTING

1¼ cups powdered sugar

1 teaspoon vanilla extract

¼ cup pure maple syrup, or as needed

1. To make the doughnuts: Preheat the oven to 375°F. Generously grease 6 mini Bundt or mini angel food cake pans or 6 muffin pan cups.

2. In a mixing bowl, stir the flour blend, xanthan gum, gelatin, baking powder, baking soda, salt, cinnamon, cloves, nutmeg, and allspice. Set aside.

3. In another bowl, combine the egg,

brown sugar, juice concentrate, maple syrup, applesauce, yogurt, and oil. Add the dry ingredients and stir just until moistened.

4. Divide the batter in half. Spoon half of the batter into the prepared pans, using about 2 generous tablespoons per pan mold.

5. Bake for 15 to 20 minutes, or until the tops spring back when touched lightly. Loosen the edges of the doughnuts and turn out onto a wire rack to cool. Wipe the pans with paper towels, grease again, and fill with the remaining batter. Bake for 15 to 20 minutes.

6. To make the frosting: Combine all the ingredients in a small bowl, adding more maple syrup, if needed, to bring frosting to spreading consistency. Dip the shaped (underside) of each doughnut into the frosting and place on waxed paper until the frosting has set.

Per doughnut

CALORIES: 315 FAT: 6g PROTEIN: 3g CARBOHYDRATES: 67g SODIUM: 307mg CHOLESTEROL: 15mg FIBER: 1g

■ ■ ■

Blueberry-Lemon Muffins

The combination of lemon and fresh blueberries is delightful. Next summer, plan ahead and freeze fresh blueberries when they're plentiful, then toss them still frozen into the batter just before spooning the batter into the muffin cups. You may need to increase the baking time by five minutes if you use frozen blueberries.

MAKES 12 MUFFINS

MUFFINS

2⅓ cups flour blend (page 11)

⅔ cup sugar

2½ teaspoons baking powder

1½ teaspoons xanthan gum

1 teaspoon unflavored gelatin powder

1 teaspoon salt

1 cup milk (cow, rice, or soy)

¼ cup canola oil

2 large eggs

1 teaspoon vanilla extract

2 teaspoons grated lemon zest

1¼ cups blueberries

GLAZE

2 tablespoons powdered sugar

2 tablespoons lemon juice

1. To make the muffins: Preheat the oven to 400°F. Grease a 12-cup standard muffin pan or use paper liners.

2. Mix the flour blend, sugar, baking powder, xanthan gum, gelatin, and salt in a large bowl with an electric mixer on low speed. Add the milk, oil, eggs, vanilla, and lemon zest and blend on medium speed until the ingredients are thoroughly moistened. Gently stir in the blueberries. Spoon the batter into the prepared muffin cups.

3. Bake for 25 minutes, or until the tops of the muffins are lightly browned.

4. To make the glaze: Combine the sugar and lemon juice in a small bowl. Drizzle over the warm muffins. Serve warm.

Per muffin

CALORIES: 280 FAT: 7g PROTEIN: 4g CARBOHYDRATES: 55g SODIUM: 274mg CHOLESTEROL: 33mg FIBER: 1g

■ ■ ■

Raspberry Muffins

If you can't find fresh raspberries, substitute frozen ones, but don't thaw them first. Just add them while they're still frozen and bake the muffins a little longer. These muffins are full of flavor and make a wonderful addition to a special brunch.

MAKES 12 MUFFINS

MUFFINS

1 ½ cups flour blend (page 11)

1 ½ teaspoons xanthan gum

⅔ cup packed light brown sugar

2 teaspoons baking powder

¼ teaspoon salt

1 teaspoon ground cinnamon

1 egg, lightly beaten

⅓ cup canola oil

½ cup milk (cow, rice, or soy)

1 teaspoon grated lemon zest

1 ¼ cups fresh raspberries

STREUSEL TOPPING

¼ cup brown rice flour

½ cup packed light brown sugar

1 teaspoon ground cinnamon

¼ cup chopped pecans

1 tablespoon canola oil

1. Preheat the oven to 350°F. Grease 12 standard muffin pan cups or use paper liners.

2. To make the muffins: Combine all the ingredients, except the raspberries, in a large mixing bowl. Mix with an electric mixer on medium speed until thoroughly blended. Gently stir in the raspberries. Pour the batter into the prepared muffin cups.

3. To make the topping: Combine all the ingredients in a small bowl. Sprinkle over the batter in each muffin cup.

4. Bake for 20 to 25 minutes, or until the muffins are lightly browned. Serve warm.

Per muffin

CALORIES: 260 FAT: 9g PROTEIN: 2g CARBOHYDRATES: 45g SODIUM: 60mg CHOLESTEROL: 15mg FIBER: 1.5g

■ ■ ■

11. | Gluten-Free Menus

"What's for dinner?" For the cook, this means not only deciding on the entrée but also choosing other dishes that taste good and look good alongside the entrée on your plate. These decisions are hard, but for the gluten-free cook they're even more challenging, especially if you're just starting out on the diet or not too familiar with cooking.

To help make your job easier, I've included dinner menus for two weeks. These menus represent a variety of different types of dishes that have compatible flavors, complement one another, look appealing on your plate, and, above all, taste good.

Perhaps this is a good time to mention the virtues of menu planning. Weekly menus help you prepare grocery lists and operate more efficiently in the kitchen because you can plan ahead, perhaps using that leftover roast chicken in a potpie or chopping enough fresh vegetables to last two days rather than one. And because you're planning how to use all of the food you buy, you cut down on waste and might actually save money.

Gluten-Free Dinners: A Two-Week Plan

Best-Ever Meat Loaf	Pork Chops with Maple Glaze
Scalloped Potatoes	Baked Acorn Squash*
Green Peas in Cream Sauce	Rice Pilaf with Dried Fruits and Nuts
Biscuits	French Bread
Chocolate Brownies	Chocolate Pudding
Lemon Chicken	Oven-Baked Crab Cakes
Steamed Asparagus*	Lettuce with Citrus Dressing
White Rice*	Buttered Corn*
Clafouti	French Bread
	Banana Cream Pie
Mexican Beef Pie	Smoked Pork Chops*
Raw Vegetable Sticks*	Potato Pancakes
Cornbread	Applesauce*
Chocolate Chip Cookies	Spiced Red Cabbage*
	Spice Cake
Cornish Game Hens with Fruit Glaze	Mexican Tortilla Casserole
Lettuce Wedges with Raspberry Vinaigrette	Lettuce with Southwestern Dressing
Steamed Broccoli*	Southwestern Beans
Herbed Brown Rice	Mexican Rice
Butterscotch Pudding	Natillas
Stir-Fried Ginger Beef with Rice	Spareribs with Chile Glaze
Fruit Salad*	Coleslaw*
Popovers	Boston Baked Beans

(continued)

Gluten-Free Dinners: A Two-Week Plan

Fresh Cantaloupe with Cinnamon*	Cornbread
	Ice Cream and Vanilla Wafers
Coq au Vin	Salmon with Asian Sauce
Tossed Salad*	Fruit Salad*
French Bread	Linguine with Pine Nuts
Yellow Cake	Easy Chocolate Cheesecake
Eggplant Parmesan	Shrimp Creole with White Rice
Lettuce with Herb Vinaigrette	Lettuce with Herb Vinaigrette
Steamed Asparagus*	Green Peas*
Bread Sticks	French Bread
Biscotti	Cheesecake with Blueberries

*These dishes are not included in this book.

More Gluten-Free Menus

If these menus leave you yearning for more, the remainder of this chapter contains 100 menus organized into the following categories.

- Quick & Easy Dinners
- Reduced-Fat, Low-Calorie Meals
- Fish & Seafood Menus
- Beef & Pork Menus
- Poultry Menus
- Southwestern Menus
- Meatless Meals

An asterisk indicates the recipe is not included in this book; however, it either requires minimal preparation, such as steaming, or it is easily found in traditional, nongluten-free cookbooks.

You should consult with your physician or nutritionist for specific dietary information about maintaining a well-balanced diet.

Quick & Easy Dinners *Ten or Fewer Ingredients; Minimal Last-Minute Preparations*	
CHICKEN	**FISH**
Cornish Game Hens with Fruit Glaze	Oven-Baked Crab Cakes
Fruit Salad*	Carrots in Maple Syrup*
Steamed Broccoli*	Whipped Potatoes*
Herbed Brown Rice	Bananas with Rum Sauce
Butterscotch Pudding	
Grilled Chicken with Ancho Chile Sauce	Red Snapper in Parchment
Orange Slices	Lettuce with Citrus Dressing
Mexican Rice	Green Beans*
Corn Bread	White Rice*
Mexican Flan	Fresh Cantaloupe with Cinnamon*
Chicken with Spicy Glaze	Orange Roughy in Parchment
Fruit Salad*	Lettuce with Buttermilk Dressing
Steamed Snow Peas*	Broiled Tomatoes*
White Rice*	White Rice*
Butterscotch Pudding	Pineapple Upside-Down Cake

(continued)

CHICKEN	FISH
Grilled Chicken with Teriyaki Glaze	Salmon with Asian Sauce
Steamed Snow Peas*	Fruit Salad*
White Rice*	Linguine with Pine Nuts
Yellow Cake with Strawberries	Easy Chocolate Cheesecake
Grilled Chipotle Chicken	Salmon with Maple Glaze
Lettuce with Lime-Cilantro Dressing	Jicama and Mandarin Oranges*
Baked Potato*	Broiled Tomatoes*
Corn Bread	Oven-Fried Potatoes
Mexican Flan	Lemon Bars
Lemon Chicken	Red Snapper with Tomato-Lime Salsa
Steamed Asparagus*	Steamed Broccoli*
White Rice*	Linguine with Pine Nuts
Clafouti	Butterscotch Pudding
Tarragon-Dijon Chicken	White Clam Sauce with Linguine
Spinach Salad with Fruit*	Lettuce with Citrus Dressing
Carrots in Maple Syrup*	Steamed Asparagus*
Herbed Rice	White Rice*
Easy Chocolate Cheesecake	Vanilla Custard
Thai Chicken	Southwestern Crab Cakes
Lettuce with Asian Vinaigrette	Lettuce with Southwestern Dressing
Asian Soba Noodles	Buttered Corn*
Broiled Tomatoes*	Sopaipillas with Honey
Cherry-Apricot Crisp	Butterscotch Pudding

(continued)

MISCELLANEOUS	MEAT
Bean Soup*	Pork Chops with Maple Glaze
Raw Vegetable Sticks*	Baked Acorn Squash*
Fennel Bread	Rice Pilaf with Dried Fruits and Nuts
Clafouti	French Bread
	Chocolate Pudding
Cheese Soup	Pork with Apples and Cabbage
Raw Vegetable Sticks*	Green Beans*
Pumpernickel Bread	Russian Black Bread
Fresh Fruit*	Ice Cream with Fresh Fruit*

Reduced-Fat, Low-Calorie Meals
400 Calories or Less per Serving; 35% Calories from Fat

Cod Baked with Vegetables	Salmon and Vegetables in Parchment
White Rice*	Herbed Brown Rice
Steamed Broccoli*	Popovers
Dilly Bread	Fresh Fruit with Vanilla Wafers
Bananas with Rum Sauce*	
Red Snapper in Parchment	Red Snapper with Tomato-Lime Salsa
Green Beans*	Green Peas*
Saffron Rice Pilaf	Homemade Egg Pasta Noodles
Green Salad*	Poached Pears*
Pavlova*	

(continued)

Reduced-Fat, Low-Calorie Meals
400 Calories or Less per Serving; 35% Calories from Fat

Grilled Chicken with Spicy Glaze	Tarragon-Dijon Chicken
Orange and Avocado Salad*	Spinach Salad*
Steamed Snow Peas*	Green Peas and Pearl Onions*
Corn Bread	Rice Pilaf with Fruits and Nuts
Clafouti	Broiled Pineapple*
Coq au Vin	Grilled Chicken with Peach Salsa
Tossed Salad*	Steamed Asparagus*
French Bread	White Rice*
Yellow Cake	Baked Apples*
Lemon-Tarragon Chicken	Thai Chicken
Steamed Green Beans*	Fruit Salad*
Breadsticks	Creamed Corn
Chocolate Cake	White Rice*
	Sponge Cake with Fruit

Fish & Seafood
Limited Spices; Fairly Mild Flavors

Cod Baked with Vegetables	Salmon and Vegetables in Parchment
Lettuce with Hazelnut Vinaigrette	Lettuce with Herb Vinaigrette
Steamed Broccoli*	Carrots in Maple Syrup*
White Rice*	Popovers
Dilly Bread	Biscotti
Banana Cream Pie	

(continued)

Fish & Seafood
Limited Spices; Fairly Mild Flavors

Sole in White Dill Sauce	Oven-Baked Crab Cakes
Snow Peas with Butter*	Lettuce with Citrus Dressing
White Rice*	Buttered Corn*
Popovers	French Bread
Coconut Cream Pie	Banana Cream Pie

Grilled Grouper with Apricot Sauce	Crab Zucchini Casserole
Lettuce with Pine Nut Dressing	Lettuce with Herb Vinaigrette
Broiled Tomatoes*	French Bread
Saffron Rice Pilaf	Cherry-Apricot Crisp
Cheesecake	

New England Clam Chowder	Orange Roughy in Parchment
Fresh Vegetable Plate*	Fruit Salad*
Dilly Bread	Broiled Tomatoes*
Boston Cream Pie	Risotto with Mushrooms and Herbs
	Butterscotch Pudding

White Clam Sauce with Linguine	Grilled Yellowfin Tuna*
Lettuce with Pine Nut Dressing	Lettuce with Avocado Dressing
Focaccia	Baked Potatoes*
Crepes with Fresh Fruit	Green Peas*
	Yellow Cake

(continued)

Bolder Flavors; Hotter Spices	
Salmon with Asian Sauce	Salmon with Tomatillo-Apple Salsa
Fruit Salad*	Lettuce with Southwestern Dressing
Asian Soba Noodles	White Rice*
Steamed Asparagus*	Sautéed Zucchini*
Vanilla Wafers	Clafouti
Shrimp Creole with White Rice	Salmon with Maple Glaze
Lettuce with Herb Vinaigrette	Lettuce with Asian Vinaigrette
Green Peas*	Oven-Fried Potatoes
French Bread	Carrots in Maple Syrup*
Cheesecake with Blueberries	Carrot Cake
Halibut with Honey Mustard Sauce	Southwestern Crab Cakes with Avocado Chile Sauce
Lettuce with Citrus Dressing	Jicama, Orange, and Avocado Salad*
French Bread	Flour Tortillas
Boston Cream Pie	Mexican Flan
Shrimp Curry	Halibut with Papaya Salsa
Steamed Snow Peas*	Lettuce with Citrus Dressing
White Rice*	Broiled Tomatoes*
Coconut Cream Pie	Baked Potatoes*
	Lemon Pudding
Cajun Shrimp on Noodles	Red Snapper and Tomato-Lime Salsa
Lettuce with Asian Dressing	Lettuce with Red Chile Dressing
Buttered Corn*	Steamed Broccoli*
French Bread	White Rice*
Yellow Cake with Strawberries	Butterscotch Pudding

Beef & Pork
Few Spices; Mild Flavors

Best-Ever Meat Loaf	Pork Chops in Mushroom Sauce
Scalloped Potatoes	Lettuce with Walnut Oil Vinaigrette
Green Peas in Cream Sauce	Broiled Tomatoes*
Biscuits	White Rice*
Chocolate Brownies	Pineapple Upside-Down Cake
Beef Paprikás with Egg Noodles	Baked Ham with Wine Sauce
Lettuce with Herb Vinaigrette	Fruit Salad*
Steamed Broccoli*	Whipped Potatoes*
Russian Black Bread	Creamed Corn
Chocolate Cake	Vanilla Custard
Sloppy Joes	Swedish Meatballs
Hamburger Buns	Homemade Egg Pasta Noodles
Carrot Sticks*	Green Peas*
Potato Chips*	Pumpernickel Bread
Chocolate Wafer Cookies	Gingerbread with Lemon Sauce
Grilled Pork Chops*	Pork Tenderloin with Brandy Sauce
Spinach Salad with Fruit	Lettuce and Pear Salad*
Butternut Squash*	Herbed Brown Rice
Spiced Red Crab Apples*	Sautéed Fennel*
Flourless Chocolate Almond Cake	Easy Chocolate Cheesecake *(continued)*

Beef & Pork
Few Spices; Mild Flavors

Roast Beef*	Smoked Pork Chops*
Baked Acorn Squash*	Potato Pancakes
Green Peas with Pearl Onions*	Applesauce*
Dilly Bread	Spiced Red Cabbage*
Chocolate Soufflé	Spice Cake

Several Spices; Bolder Flavors

Pork Chops with Mustard Sauce	Pork Ribs with Maple Glaze
Fruit Salad*	Coleslaw*
Sautéed Zucchini*	Boston Baked Beans
Whipped Potatoes*	Baked Potatoes*
Shortbread with Sliced Fruit	Rhubarb Meringue Dessert

Pork Chops with Apples and Cabbage	Pork Tenderloin with Apple Chutney
Steamed Green Beans*	Lettuce with Walnut Oil Vinaigrette
Fennel Bread	Brussels Sprouts in Walnut Oil*
Gingerbread with Lemon Sauce	Linguine with Pine Nuts
	Cream Puffs

Mexican Beef Pie	Stir-Fried Ginger Beef with Rice
Raw Vegetable Sticks*	Fruit Salad*
Corn Bread	Popovers
Chocolate Chip Cookies	Fresh Cantaloupe with Cinnamon* *(continued)*

Several Spices; Bolder Flavors

White Bean Cassoulet with Sausage	Spareribs with Chile Glaze
Lettuce with Herb Vinaigrette	Coleslaw*
Bread Sticks	Boston Baked Beans
Chocolate Cake	Corn Bread
	Ice Cream and Vanilla Wafers
Pork Chops with Red Wine Sauce	Spaghetti and Meatballs
Lettuce and Pear Salad*	Green Salad with Herb Vinaigrette
Steamed Broccoli*	French Bread
White Rice*	Chocolate Brownies
Lemon Pudding	

Poultry
Few Spices; Mild Flavors

Chicken Paprikás	Oven-Fried Chicken
Green Beans*	Green Peas with Pearl Onions*
Homemade Egg Pasta Noodles	Hash-Brown Casserole
French Bread	Biscuits
Chocolate Pudding	Apple Pie*
Creamed Chicken on Biscuits	Oven-Fried Chicken
Fresh Fruit*	Potato Salad*
Steamed Asparagus*	Boston Baked Beans
Gingersnaps	Biscuits
	Watermelon* *(continued)*

Poultry
Few Spices; Mild Flavors

Lemon Chicken	Tarragon-Dijon Chicken
Steamed Asparagus*	Mixed Green Salad*
White Rice*	Green Peas*
Cream Puffs	Herbed Brown Rice
	Lemon Pudding
Chicken Shepherd's Pie	Roast Chicken*
Lettuce with Hazelnut Vinaigrette	Waldorf Salad*
Fruit Salad with Balsamic Dressing*	Creamed Corn
French Bread	Baked Potatoes*
Boston Cream Pie	Dilly Bread
	Cherry Pie*
Chicken and Broccoli Quiche	Chicken Breasts with Mushrooms
Fruit Salad*	Risotto with Mushrooms and Herbs
French Bread	Carrots in Maple Syrup*
Carrot Cake	French Bread
	Pavlova*

More Spices; Bolder Flavors

Chicken Tandoori	Grilled Chicken with Peach Salsa
Cucumber Salad*	Lettuce with Avocado Dressing
Curried Rice Pilaf with Raisins	Green Peas*
Popovers	French Bread
Fresh Blueberries*	Pineapple Upside-Down Cake

(continued)

More Spices; Bolder Flavors

Chicken Curry	Chicken Cacciatore on Noodles
Green Peas*	Lettuce with Buttermilk Dressing
White Rice*	Brussels Sprouts in Walnut Oil
French Bread	Popovers
Fruit Plate with Berry Sauce*	Chocolate Cake
Grilled Chicken with Spicy Glaze	Chicken Curry
Sautéed Fennel	Steamed Broccoli*
Spinach Salad*	Saffron Rice Pilaf
Clafouti	Poached Pears*
Coq au Vin	Thai Chicken
Lettuce with Herb Vinaigrette	Ambrosia Salad*
Green Peas*	Green Peas*
French Bread	Asian Soba Noodles
Chocolate Cake	Pavlova*
Grilled Chicken with Teriyaki Glaze	Spicy Oven-Fried Chicken
Mixed Green Salad*	Waldorf Salad*
Orange-Glazed Carrots*	Creamed Corn
Wild Rice with Dried Fruit	Oven-Fried Potatoes
Lemon Pudding	Biscuits
	Gingerbread with Lemon Sauce

Southwestern Menus

Grilled Chicken and Ancho Chiles	Chicken Burritos* with Sauces:
Black Bean Salad*	Red Chile Sauce
Buttered Corn*	Tomatillo Sauce
Biscuits	Green Chile Sauce
Vanilla Custard with Fresh Fruit*	Southwestern Beans
	Mexican Flan
Grilled Chipotle Chicken	Red Chile Barbecued Chicken
Jicama and Mandarin Oranges*	Coleslaw*
Green Peas*	Baked Potatoes*
Corn Bread	French Bread
Mexican Flan	Lemon Bars
Turkey Mole	Chile Relleno Casserole
Fresh Fruit*	Fruit Salad*
Corn Bread	Flour Tortillas
Mexican Rice	Mexican Wedding Cakes
Mexican Chocolate Cake	
Enchiladas	Mexican Chicken Casserole
Mexican Rice	Lettuce with Lime-Cilantro Dressing
Refried Beans	French Bread
Flour Tortillas	Lemon Bars
Anise–Pine Nut Cookies	

(continued)

Southwestern Menus

Grilled Chicken with Peach Salsa	Mexican Tortilla Casserole
Grapefruit and Avocado Salad*	Jicama, Orange, and Avocado Salad*
Green Peas*	Southwestern Beans
White Rice with Pine Nuts*	Corn Bread
Coconut Macaroons	Natillas

Meatless Meals

Huevos Rancheros	Veggieburgers
Fresh Fruit*	Hamburger Buns
Refried Beans	Carrot Sticks*
Mexican Wedding Cakes	Oven-Fried Potatoes
	Butterscotch Pudding
Mexican Tortilla Casserole	Eggplant Parmesan
Lettuce with Southwestern Dressing	Lettuce with Herb Vinaigrette
Southwestern Beans	Steamed Asparagus*
Mexican Rice	Bread Sticks
Natillas	Biscotti

Appendix: Wheat-Free Flours & Dairy Substitutes

Wheat-Flour Equivalents for Baking

Remember that you will rarely use any of these flours alone. They are usually blended with other gluten-free flours for the best results. Flours from reputable sources will usually measure consistently, although differences in flour milling processes by different companies may affect the texture. As you become more experienced with these flours, you'll be able to judge if the dough is too dry, too moist, or just right.

Use the following amounts of flour in place of 1 cup wheat flour.

KIND OF FLOUR	AMOUNT
Amaranth	1 cup
Arrowroot	1 cup
Bean (garbanzo/fava bean)	1 cup
Buckwheat	⅞ cup
Corn	1 cup

(continued)

KIND OF FLOUR	AMOUNT
Cornmeal	¾ cup
Cornstarch	¾ cup
Garbanzo (chickpea)	¾ cup
Indian rice grass (Montina)	1 cup
Millet	1 cup
Nuts (any kind, finely ground)	½ cup
Potato starch	¾ cup
Quinoa	1 cup
Rice (brown or white)	⅞ cup
Sago starch	¾ cup
Sorghum	1 cup
Soy	½ cup + ½ cup potato starch
Sweet rice	⅞ cup
Tapioca flour or starch	1 cup
Teff	⅞ cup

Substitutes for Wheat as a Thickener

Many of us learned to cook using wheat flour as a thickener in gravies, soups, and sauces. Other starches and flours can thicken certain foods, but each alternative has certain strengths and weaknesses, so use the following information to choose among them.

In place of 1 tablespoon wheat flour, use the following.

INGREDIENT AND SUGGESTED AMOUNT	TRAITS	SUGGESTED USES
Agar (Kanten) 1½ teaspoons	Follow package directions. Colorless and flavorless. Sets at room temperature. Gels acidic liquids. Thin sauces need less.	Puddings, pie fillings, gelatin desserts, ice creams, glazes, cheese: holds moisture and improves texture in pastry products.
Amaranth starch 1½ teaspoons	Dissolve in cold water before using.	Puddings, pie fillings, and sauces: available from www.nuworldamaranth.com
Arrowroot 1½ teaspoons	Mix with cold liquid before using. Thickens at lower temperature than wheat flour or cornstarch, so it's better for eggs or sauces that are not boiled. Add during last 5 minutes of cooking. Serve immediately after thickening. Clear, shiny. Semisoft when cool.	Any food requiring clear, shiny sauce, but good for egg or starch dishes for which high heat is undesirable: gives appearance of oil when none is used. Don't overcook, or sauce will become thin.

(continued)

INGREDIENT AND SUGGESTED AMOUNT	TRAITS	SUGGESTED USES
Bean flour (chickpea) 1 tablespoon	Produces yellowish, rich-looking sauce.	Soups, stews, gravies: has slight bean taste.
Cornstarch 1½ teaspoons	Mix with cold liquid before using. Stir just until boiling. Makes transparent, shiny sauce. Has slightly starchy flavor. Thicker and rigid when cool.	Puddings, pie fillings, fruit sauces, soups: gives appearance of oil when none is used.
Gelatin powder (unflavored) 1½ teaspoons	Dissolve in cold water, then heat until liquid is clear before using. Won't gel acid.	Gelled puddings, aspics, cheesecakes
Guar gum 1½ teaspoons	Mix with liquid before using. Has high fiber content and may act as a laxative.	Especially good for rice-flour recipes
Sweet rice flour 1 tablespoon	Excellent thickening agent	Soups, stews, or gravies and sauces such as vegetable sauces
Rice flour (brown or white) 1 tablespoon	Mix with cold liquid before using. Has somewhat grainy texture. Hot or cold, has same consistency.	Soups, stews, or gravies
Tapioca flour 1½ tablespoons	Mix with cold or hot liquid before using. Add during last 5 minutes of cooking to avoid being rubbery. Produces transparent, shiny sauce. Thick, soft gel when cool.	Soups, stews, gravies, potato dishes

(continued)

INGREDIENT AND SUGGESTED AMOUNT	TRAITS	SUGGESTED USES
Quick-cooking tapioca (precooked) 2 teaspoons	Mix with fruit; let stand 15 minutes before baking.	Fruit pies, cobblers, and tapioca pudding
Xanthan gum 1 teaspoon	Mix with dry ingredients first, then add.	Puddings, salad dressings, and gravies

HOW I USE DIFFERENT THICKENERS

I'm often asked how I use the different thickeners in my own kitchen. For fruit pie fillings, I use quick-cooking tapioca, cornstarch, or potato starch because they make a transparent sauce that allows the beauty of the fruit to show through. For puddings, I use cornstarch or amaranth starch because they give good body and substance. For cream soups, I use sweet rice flour because it produces a creamy, opaque texture that makes the soup look richer than it really is, yet it doesn't produce so much shine that the soup looks artificial. For savory sauces used on meat or vegetables, I use cornstarch, although if only a little thickening is needed I also use a little arrowroot to give the sauce a shiny gloss that makes it look like it contains fat (when it might not have any fat at all). For salad dressings, I use xanthan gum to provide body, especially when the dressing is just blended with a whisk rather than thoroughly emulsified in a blender.

The Wonderful World of Gluten-Free Flours

This section is designed to help you better understand the different gluten-free flours in terms of baking characteristics, color, flavor, and storage.

FLOUR	BAKING	COLOR AND FLAVOR	GENERAL COMMENTS	STORAGE
Amaranth	Especially good in dark-colored baked goods or those with spices, such as chocolate cakes or cookies, spice cakes, and dark breads. Tends to brown quickly. Best when blended with other flours as no more than 15% to 20% of blend.	Mild, grainlike, nutty. Color varies from beige to nearly black but usually light tan.	Not related to wheat or other grains, it was cultivated long ago by the Aztecs. Color varies depending on origin. Higher in protein and fiber than any other grain.	Airtight container in cool, dry, dark place. Refrigeration preferred since flavor may intensify or turn rancid during prolonged storage. Buy in small quantities to avoid aging.
Arrowroot	Good for baking because it adds no flavor of its own and lightens baked goods. If used as breading, produces golden brown crust.	Snow white in color; looks like cornstarch. Flavorless.	Silky, fine powder. Often used to replace cornstarch or tapioca flour.	Airtight container in cool, dry, dark place

FLOUR	BAKING	COLOR AND FLAVOR	GENERAL COMMENTS	STORAGE
Bean	Two kinds of bean flour: (1) pure garbanzo or chickpea flour, and (2) blend of garbanzo flour and fava bean flour available from Authentic Foods, Bob's Red Mill, and Ener-G Foods. (See Mail-Order Sources, page 257). Both flours provide protein that is beneficial in baking. Use in combination with other flours to totally (or partially) replace rice flour.	Light tan or yellowish. Slight "beany" flavor, especially if flour is pure chickpea or garbanzo bean, less so if using garbanzo/fava bean combination. The latter gives slightly sweet taste to baked goods.	Adds important protein to otherwise "starchy" gluten-free flour blends.	Airtight container in cool, dry, dark place

(continued)

FLOUR	BAKING	COLOR AND FLAVOR	GENERAL COMMENTS	STORAGE
Chestnut Flour	Lends a silky texture and nutty flavor. Don't confuse it with water-chestnut flour, which is quite starchy. Should be used with other flours (up to 25% of the blend in baking).	Ground from chestnuts, this is a light beige flour.	Also called *marrons*, chestnuts are lower in fat than other nuts.	Store in dark, dry place.
Corn	Excellent in corn bread, muffins, and waffles, especially when blended with cornmeal. (This is not cornmeal, but finely ground corn flour.)	Light yellow in color. Tastes like corn.	Smooth flour from corn	Airtight container in cool, dry, dark place

FLOUR	BAKING	COLOR AND FLAVOR	GENERAL COMMENTS	STORAGE
Cornmeal	Excellent in corn bread, muffins, and waffles, especially when blended with corn flour. Blue cornmeal can be substiuted in muffins and waffles.	White or yellow. Tastes like corn. Blue cornmeal is grayish blue and has a somewhat stronger flavor.	Coarser than corn flour; often used in Mexican dishes. Used in polenta but is often a coarser grind than regular cornmeal. Blue cornmeal can substitute for white or yellow cornmeal in some Mexican dishes.	Airtight container in cool, dry, dark place
Millet	Lends a light-yellow tint to baked goods and produces a light, dry crumb with a smooth, thin crust. Millet performs best when blended with other flours, comprising no more than 25% of the flour blend.	Light yellow color with mild, slightly cornlike flavor	Very high in protein, but due to its high alkalinity, it is one of the easier grains to digest.	Refrigerate, tightly covered, for two months. Purchase millet flour in small amounts and use it quickly because it can become bitter and rancid.

(continued)

FLOUR	BAKING	COLOR AND FLAVOR	GENERAL COMMENTS	STORAGE
Montina Indian rice grass	Relatively high in protein, it works best blended with other, lighter flours. Use as 25% of the flour blend.	Light brown/gray color. Produces darker-colored baked goods with a hearty "wheatlike" flavor and pleasant "chew" due to higher fiber content.	This flour was developed from Indian rice grass that is grown in Montana.	Store in cool, dry, dark place, or refrigerate, tightly covered.
Potato	Use in very small quantities in baking; adds crispness and density or "tooth" to baked goods.	Heavy, light tan flour made from whole potatoes, including the skins. Slight potato flavor.	Often mistaken for potato starch but performs quite differently in baking.	Airtight container in refrigerator to prevent rancidity
Potato Starch	Excellent baking properties, especially when combined with eggs. Lumps easily, so stir with whisk before measuring.	Very white, fine powder. Bland flavor.	Very fine, powdery texture. Made from the dried starch of potatoes. Not the same as potato flour, which is made from dried and ground whole potatoes. Potato flour is heavy and used very little in wheat-free cooking.	Airtight container in cool, dry, dark place

FLOUR	BAKING	COLOR AND FLAVOR	GENERAL COMMENTS	STORAGE
Quinoa	Excellent in all types of baking, including cakes, cookies, breads, and biscuits. Best if blended with other flours (no more than 25%) and used in highly spiced or flavored foods.	Grain looks like sesame seeds. Flour color ranges from hues of red/yellow/orange to pink/purple/black, although flour tends to be tan. Flavor is somewhat nutty and can dominate baked goods.	Not actually a cereal grain but a member of the Chenopodiaceae family (related to beets and spinach). It is a complete protein and originally grown by the Incas of Peru.	Airtight container in cool, dry, dark place. Keeps well.
Rice (white or brown)	A bit gritty by itself, but works fine when combined with other flours. Should be about two-thirds of total flour blend. The coarser the grind, the more liquid needed.	White rice flour is white; brown rice flour has slight tan tint. Bland, pleasant-tasting flavor.	Milled from broken hulls of rice kernels. Among least "allergenic" of all flours. Mostly starch and nutritionally inferior since bran and germ layers have been removed in milling.	Airtight container in cool, dry, dark place. Refrigerate brown rice flour to avoid rancidity.

(continued)

FLOUR	BAKING	COLOR AND FLAVOR	GENERAL COMMENTS	STORAGE
Sorghum	Works very well in all kinds of baking, especially bread. Best if blended with other flours, but can comprise up to half of flour blend.	Light tan color. Fairly bland flavor, although some people liken its flavor to that of wheat.	Newer, table sorghum variety is grown for human consumption (also called white-food sorghum).	Store in airtight container in dark, dry, cool place.
Soy	Excellent. Works well in baked goods with nuts, fruits, or chocolate. Best when combined with other flours, such as rice.	Yellow in color. Bland, somewhat nutty flavor—leans toward "beany." Flavor can be camouflaged by mixing with spices, fruit, nuts, or chocolate.	Makes crispy coating for breading. Higher in protein and fat than other flours. Short shelf life, so purchase in small amounts to avoid spoilage. A common allergen, so use soy cautiously.	Airtight container in cool, dry, dark place. Best if refrigerated.
Sweet Potato	Produces baked goods with a great taste and texture. Its faint sweetness, however, will affect gravies and other savory sauces.	Light orange-yellow–colored flour with a faintly sweet taste	Ground from sweet potatoes, this hard-to-find flour is available in some specialty stores and at www.ener-g.com. Sweet potatoes, a member of the morning glory family, are one of the least allergenic foods on earth.	Refrigerate, tightly covered.

FLOUR	BAKING	COLOR AND FLAVOR	GENERAL COMMENTS	STORAGE
Sweet Rice	Manufacturers suggest using it in muffins, breads, and cakes although some sources recommend using only small amounts. Adds a nice elasticity to baked goods.	White, bland in flavor. Easily confused with white rice flour because they look alike.	Sometimes called sticky rice; often used in Chinese cooking. Contains more starch than rice flours, making it an excellent thickener. Helps inhibit separation of sauces when they're chilled or frozen.	Airtight container in cool, dark, dry place
Tapioca	Excellent in baked products when it makes up 25% to 50% of total flour. Lightens baked goods and imparts "chewiness" to breads. Browns quickly and produces crispy coating in breading.	Snow-white, velvety powder. Bland flavor	Sometimes called cassava or cassava starch. Similar to arrowroot and can be used interchangeably.	Airtight container in cool, dark, dry place

(continued)

FLOUR	BAKING	COLOR AND FLAVOR	GENERAL COMMENTS	STORAGE
Teff	A little gritty, but works well in baked goods such as cakes or breads if used as 25% to 50% of total flour. Best in "dark" baked goods such as chocolate cake or brownies, pumpernickel bread, or gingerbread.	Brown color. Slightly strong-tasting.	Belongs to a tribe of its own in the grain family.	Airtight container in cool, dark, dry place

Hidden Sources of Gluten

The following list contains those foods or ingredients that are often suspicious. This list is based on the latest information from gluten-free experts, but manufacturing practices can change, ingredients can be modified, or new ingredients can be introduced to previously safe foods. So, to put a new slant on an old phrase, it's "eater beware." As always, the responsibility for what you eat lies with you. If you have any doubts about a food, don't eat it!

It is also important to note that any food can be a problem to certain people, regardless of whether they have celiac disease or not. You can have food sensitivities in addition to celiac disease. So, just because you have a reaction to a certain food does not mean that food contains gluten.

- *Beverages:* Distilled liquors, such as scotch, whiskey, or bourbon, do not contain gluten because the gluten peptides cannot survive the distillation process. However, beverages such as beer and ale are fermented rather than distilled and contain gluten from the barley or wheat from which they are made. Wine is made from grapes and does not contain gluten. Unless you know the source of the flavor, beware of any alcoholic beverage (even if it is presumed to be safe, such as vodka) if it has flavorings added after distillation. Some hard ciders are gluten-free, because they are made from fermented fruit.

  Nonalcoholic beverages such as Postum and Ovaltine contain gluten.
- *Breads:* Unless the label says "gluten-free," avoid any biscuits, breads, crackers, croutons, crumbs, doughnuts, tortillas, or wafers. Avoid breads made of spelt, kamut, barley, rye, and triticale. Words on the label that indicate wheat include *semolina, durum, white flour, unbleached flour,* and *all-purpose flour.*
- *Brown rice syrup:* This can be made from barley; however, Lundberg Brown Rice Syrup is gluten-free.
- *Candy:* Wheat may be used to prevent sticking during the shaping or handling of candy. Wheat may also be an ingredient in candy, such as licorice, to give it body.
- *Canola oil:* This healthy oil is made from a new variety of rapeseed called canola seed. It is gluten-free.
- *Caramel color:* This *may* contain malt syrup or wheat starch, if the product is foreign-made. In the U.S., caramel color is most likely made from corn, because corn

makes a better product and the only two manufacturers of caramel color in the U.S. use corn.

■ *Cereal:* Avoid those made from wheat, rye, barley, spelt, and kamut or cereals that contain malt flavoring or malt syrup. Oats are naturally gluten-free but may be contaminated with wheat, so it's best to avoid oat cereals as well. There is an increasing array of cereals made from corn, rice, buckwheat, sorghum, quinoa, and amaranth, so you still have plenty of choices.

■ *Citric acid:* This is always a suspicious ingredient since citric acid can be fermented from corn, beets, molasses, or wheat. While corn is the only source used by manufacturers in the U.S., about 25% of the citric acid used in food and drink in the U.S. is imported from other countries and could contain wheat. By the way, Coke and Pepsi use corn in their citric acid.

■ *Coffee:* Pure coffee is gluten-free, but some flavored coffees may use wheat as a flavor carrier. Make sure that instant coffee is just pure coffee, without wheat as a filler. Labels on coffee substitutes, such as those made from grains, should be read carefully.

■ *Condiments and baking ingredients:* Wheat-free tamari soy sauce is gluten-free. Pure spices are gluten-free, but some spice mixes may contain wheat as a filler. Lea and Perrins Worcestershire sauce is gluten-free in the U.S. but not in Canada. Coleman's dry mustard contains wheat, so grind your own mustard seeds or use Durkee or Spice Island. Condiments such as ketchup and mustard, which were previously off-limits because of the distilled vinegar, are usually gluten-free unless the label lists a gluten-containing ingredient. Check labels on all condiments to be safe.

■ *Dairy products:* Some flavored or low-fat yogurts contain modified food starch (which is probably corn, especially if it's made in the U.S., but could be wheat). Look for the source of the modified food starch on the label, or choose yogurts with pectin (fruit-based). Malted milk, processed cheese spread, low-fat or light sour cream, and chocolate milk may contain wheat.

■ *Desserts and other sweets:* Avoid commercial pudding mixes, some cake decorations, and marzipan. Look for the words *gluten-free* on the label of commercially baked goods.

■ *Dextrin:* In the U.S., it is usually made from corn or tapioca. But it can be made from wheat, so avoid this ingredient

■ *Distilled vinegar:* Experts believe that gluten cannot survive the distillation process, so grain-based vinegars (except malt vinegar) are considered gluten-free. (See

Gluten-Free Living magazine, Sept./Oct. 1999 and Volume 8, no. 3, 2003.) Malt vinegar has malt flavor from barley added in after distillation. Wine, rice, or cider vinegar are still good choices for the gluten-free diet. If flavorings or seasonings are added to the vinegar, check the label for ingredients.

■ *Flavorings:* Generally speaking, natural flavorings are gluten-free. However, natural flavorings used in or on meats may contain gluten, since wheat has a natural affinity for meat and meat products.

■ *Grains:* The "new" grains such as amaranth, buckwheat, sorghum, quinoa, and teff are gluten-free. In most cases, these grains are not even botanically related to wheat.

■ *Hydrolyzed vegetable protein:* The word *vegetable* can mean anything. Since 1993, this ingredient can't appear on a food label. However, it may still be possible to find old foods that still bear this ingredient. Today, the ingredient would be labeled with its source, such as hydrolyzed soy protein.

■ *Malt:* Malt is made from barley and therefore contains gluten.

■ *Maltodextrin:* In the U.S., maltodextrin is made from corn, rice, or potato. It cannot be made from gluten unless it is declared on the ingredient label. So, unless your product is foreign-made, the maltodextrin should not contain gluten. (See *Gluten-Free Living* magazine, Volume 8, no. 2, 2003 for a fuller explanation.)

■ *Meat, fish, and eggs:* Avoid any meat that's been breaded or in which fillers might be used, such as sausage, luncheon meats, or hot dogs. Avoid self-basting turkeys. Buy tuna packed in spring water rather than oil. Egg substitutes are not necessarily pure eggs and contain many additional ingredients, such as wheat.

■ *Modified food starch:* Usually made from corn when it is used in food, it could be made from wheat or some other food, especially if the food product was produced outside the U.S. The content of the modified food starch should be declared on the label. The word *starch* usually means cornstarch. However, when starch is used in pharmaceuticals, these rules may not apply.

■ *Mono and diglycerides:* These are fats and not a concern in their liquid state. If they are used in their dry form, then wheat might be used. However, wheat is declared on the label by the two major food manufacturers, Kraft and General Mills.

■ *Pastas:* Look for "gluten-free" on the label. You can eat Asian rice noodles, bean threads, and commercial pasta made from pure buckwheat or those made from corn, quinoa, potato starch, or rice.

■ *Soups and chowders:* Many canned soups, soup mixes, and bouillon cubes or granules contain wheat as a thickener or filler.

- *Seasonings:* These are usually made from combinations of herbs and spices and may have a carrier such as wheat flour, which may or may not be declared.

- *Soy sauce:* Always look for wheat-free tamari soy sauce, because regular soy sauce is made with wheat.

- *Spices:* A pure spice that has only one name (e.g., cinnamon) is made from cinnamon only. If there is no ingredient label, then the cinnamon is pure cinnamon with no additives or fillers.

- *Textured soy protein (TSP)* and *textured vegetable protein (TVP):* These are usually made from soy, not wheat.

- *Vanilla:* Vanilla is now known to be gluten-free because gluten cannot survive the distillation process. (See *Gluten-Free Living* magazine, Nov./Dec. 1999.) If in doubt, look for gluten-free, non-alcohol flavorings.

- *Vegetables:* "Vegetable starch" or "vegetable protein" on the label could mean corn, peanuts, rice, soy, or wheat. Avoid vegetables that are breaded, creamed, or scalloped.

- *Yeast:* The baker's yeast used in breads is gluten-free. Common brands such as Red Star and Fleischman are gluten-free. Nutritional yeast (a supplement) and brewer's yeast (a by-product of the brewing industry) may or may not be gluten-free, so check with the manufacturer. Autolyzed yeast, commonly used as a food flavoring, is generally gluten-free.

To stay informed about ingredient safety, subscribe to *Gluten-Free Living* magazine, or visit websites such as www.celiac.com and www.clanthompson.com. Or purchase the Commercial Product Listing from the Celiac Sprue Association or the product listing from the Tri-County Celiac Support Group. See the Appendix for addresses.

This section is based on information from *Gluten-Free Living* magazine; the Gluten-Free Living conference by Ann Whalen, September 2003; *Quick Start Diet Guide* by the Gluten Intolerance Group and the Celiac Disease Foundation; and *Gluten-Free Diet: A Comprehensive Resource Guide, 2002,* by Shelley Case, Bs.C., R.D.

Baking with Dairy Substitutes

Although this is a gluten-free book, I also include instructions for dairy substitutes. This is because sensitivities to dairy products are likely to accompany gluten sensitivity, especially in the case of those who have celiac disease.

Milk is one of the easiest ingredients to make substitutions for in baking, although some milk substitutes impart a subtle flavor to baked goods and may affect their browning. Read labels to avoid problem ingredients such as casein, a milk protein often found in lactose-free foods. You might think that so-called dairy-free products would not contain any dairy, but they can still contain casein.

Individuals with celiac disease should also avoid rice milk made with brown rice syrup (which may be processed with barley malt) unless the safety of the brown rice syrup can be verified.

In place of 1 cup cow's milk, use:

SUBSTITUTE	AMOUNT TO USE CHARACTERISTICS	WHEN TO USE/TIPS
Rice milk (rice beverage): Be sure to buy brands that are vitamin fortified.	1 cup Mild flavor, white color. Looks like skim milk from cows.	In any recipe, although it is slightly sweet tasting. Make sure it's gluten-free.
Soy milk (soy beverage): Be sure to buy brands that are vitamin fortified.	1 cup Slight soy flavor, light tan in color. Can buy in liquid or powder form (which must be mixed with water). Powdered version makes milk with a lighter color. Unsweetened versions for savory dishes.	Best in recipes with stronger flavors so soy taste is masked, if desired, and in baked goods with darker colors, since soy milk darkens with heat. Make sure it's gluten-free.
Nut milk (usually almond): People with allergies to nuts should use caution. Ener-G NutQuik is made of almond meal and guar gum.	1 cup Mild, slightly nutty flavor Light brown color	Best in dessert recipes. Tastes slightly "off" in savory dishes.

(continued)

SUBSTITUTE	AMOUNT TO USE CHARACTERISTICS	WHEN TO USE/TIPS
Goat milk: Available in powdered and liquid form, also in low-fat liquid. Not recommended for those with true milk allergies.	1 cup Most closely resembles cow's milk in color (pure white).	In any recipe. Works especially well in ice cream, puddings, and other milk-based dishes. Aseptic and powdered varieties have stronger flavor.

DRY MILK POWDER

If the recipe calls for dry milk powder, it refers to the heavy, dense powder made by companies such as Bob's Red Mill rather than the lighter, more crystalline version made by companies such as Carnation. Many people use nondairy powders made by Better Than Milk and Solait. Check to make sure the ingredients are safe for your diet.

In place of 1 cup evaporated skim milk, use:

SUBSTITUTE	AMOUNT TO USE	WHEN TO USE/TIPS
Ener-G NutQuik or SoyQuik or other nondairy milk powders: Mix at double strength.	1 cup	Recipes with evaporated skim milk. Calories and nutrient values double. Flavor is stronger.

In place of 1 cup buttermilk, use:

SUBSTITUTE	AMOUNT TO USE	WHEN TO USE/TIPS
Use 1 tablespoon fresh lemon juice or cider vinegar or reconstituted Ener-G gluten-free vinegar and enough rice, soy, or nut milk to make 1 cup.	1 cup (Some nondairy milks produce a thinner buttermilk. If so, use 2 tablespoons less of nondairy buttermilk per cup specified in recipe.)	Any recipe calling for buttermilk

DENSITY OF MILK

Whether it's a liquid nondairy milk (called beverage) or one mixed from powder, the thinner the milk, the less you'll need. For example, reduce liquid by 1 to 2 tablespoons per cup if you use skim milk or low-fat milk in place of whole milk or if you use rice milk instead of soy milk. Liquid milk densities vary by brand, so experiment a little. The ratio of powder to water affects the density of milks made from nondairy powders.

LACTOSE-REDUCED MILK

You may use gluten-free, lactose-reduced milk in these recipes; however, you'll need to experiment to achieve the desired results.

In place of 1 cup yogurt, use:

SUBSTITUTE	AMOUNT TO USE	WHEN TO USE/TIPS
Goat yogurt (People with true milk allergy should avoid all goat products.)	1 cup	Any recipe calling for yogurt. However, tapioca in goat yogurt can make baked items "doughy."
Soy yogurt	1 cup	Not well-suited to heat but works well in dips, ice creams, and other nonbaked items. Won't drain for Yogurt Cheese (page 94).
Nondairy milk liquid	⅔ cup	Any recipe calling for yogurt. Best to add liquid in ⅓-cup increments to avoid adding too much.

CHEESE

Although there are several "nondairy" cheeses, such as Parmesan cheese made from rice, soy, or nuts, it is difficult to find one that doesn't have other problem ingredients. For example, they may contain milk proteins called calcium caseinate (e.g., Soyco's Rice Parmesan), sodium caseinate, or casein. Others include oats (which is off-limits for those with celiac). Also, plain milk may contain one set of ingredients, but flavored versions may contain a different set of ingredients.

SOUR CREAM AND CREAM CHEESE

Soyco makes a rice-based version, however, check the label to make sure it's right for your diet; the milk protein, casein, is present in both items. Soymage makes a casein-free sour cream alternative. Some sour creams may have thickeners, especially those that are low-fat, and those thickeners may include wheat. Tofutti makes a dairy-free cream cheese.

$\mathcal{R}$esources

The following is a partial list of resources for those on gluten-free diets. Ask your physician about local support groups for people with food allergies, celiac disease, or other conditions that require avoidance of gluten. This list is not intended as an endorsement of any association or organization.

Allergy and Asthma Network, Mothers of Asthmatics, Inc.
3554 Chain Ridge Rd., Suite 200
Fairfax, VA 22030-2709
800.878.4403 (help line); 703.385.4403

American Academy of Allergy, Asthma, and Immunology
611 E. Wells St.
Milwaukee, WI 53202
800.822.2762 (help line); 414.272.6071

American Celiac Society Dietary Support Coalition
P.O. Box 23455
New Orleans, LA 70183
www.amerceliacsoc@netscape.net

American Celiac Task Force
www.celiaccenter.org/taskforce.asp
e-mail: actf@fogworks.net

For e-mail updates, type "subscribe" in subject line at:
celiac_list@capwiz.mailmanager.net

American Diabetes, Inc.
1660 Duke St.
Alexandria, VA 22314
800.DIABETES; 800.232.3472
www.diabetes.org

American Dietetic Association
120 S. Riverside Plaza, Suite 2000
Chicago, IL 60606
312.899.0040
www.eatright.org

Asthma/Allergy Foundation of America
1125 15th St., N.W., Suite 502
Washington, DC 20005
800.7ASTHMA (help line)
FAX 202.466.7643

Autism Network-Diet Intervention (ANDI)
P.O. Box 335
Pennington, NJ 08534
FAX 609.737.8453
www.AutismNDI.com

Autism Resource Network
904 Main St.
Hopkins, MN 55343
952.988.0088
FAX 952.988.0099
www.autismshop.com

Autism Society of America
7910 Woodmont Ave., Suite 300
Bethesda, MD 20814-3015
800.3Autism, ext. 150; 301.657.0881
FAX 303.657.0869

Celiac Disease Center
Columbia University
630 W. 168 St., Box 118
New York, NY 10032
www.cpmcnet.columbia.edu/dept/gi/celiac.html

Celiac Disease Foundation
13251 Ventura Blvd., Suite 1
Studio City, CA 91604-1838
818.990.2354
FAX 818.990.2379
www.celiac.org/cdf

University of Chicago Celiac Disease Program
University of Chicago
5839 S. Maryland Ave., MC 4065
Chicago, IL 60637-1470
773.702.7593
FAX 773.702.0666
www.gi.bsd.uchicago.edu/diseases/nutritional/celiac_disease.html

Celiac Sprue Association/USA
P.O. Box 31700
Omaha, NE 68131-0700
877.CSA.4CSA
FAX 402.558.1347
www.csaceliacs.org

Celiac Sprue Research Foundation
P.O. Box 61193
Palo Alto, CA 94306-1193
www.celiacsupport.stanford.edu

Center for Celiac Research
University of Maryland
22 S. Greene St., Box 140
Baltimore, MD 21201
www.celiaccenter.org

Feingold Association of U.S.
P.O. Box 6550
Alexandria, VA 22306
800.321.3287
www.feingold.org

Fine, M.D., Dr. Kenneth
Intestinal Health Institute
(Website for celiac disease and other forms of gluten sensitivity)
www.enterolab.com
www.finerhealth.com

Food Allergy/Anaphylaxis Network (FAAN)
11781 Lee Jackson Hwy. #160
Fairfax, VA 22033
800.929.4040
www.foodallergy.org
fan@worldweb.net
www.fankids.org (for kids)

Friends of Celiac Disease Research
8832 N. Port Washington Rd. #204
Milwaukee, WI 53217

414.540.6679
FAX 414.540.0587
friends@aero.net

Gluten-Free Living magazine
P.O. Box 105
Hastings-on-Hudson, NY 10706
914.969.2018

Gluten Intolerance Group
15110 Tenth Ave., SW, Suite A
Seattle, WA 98166-1820
206.246.6652
FAX 206.246.6531
www.gluten.net; gig@gluten.net

Living Without magazine
P.O. Box 2126
Northbrook, IL 60065
847.480.8810
FAX 847.480.8810
www.livingwithout.com

National Attention Deficit Disorder Assoc.
1788 Second St., Suite 200
Highland Park, IL 60035
847.432.2332

National Grain Sorghum Producers
P.O. Box 5309
Lubbock, TX 79408
806.749.3478
www.sorghumgrowers.com
(info on table or white sorghum)

National Jewish Medical and Research Center
1400 Jackson St.
Denver, CO 80206
800.222.5864 (lung line); 303.388.4461
www.njc.org

Tri-County Celiac Support Group
47819 Vistas Circle
Canton, MI 48788
(gluten-free product list)

York Nutritional Laboratories
2700 N. 29 Ave., Suite 205
Hollywood, FL 33020
888.751.3388
FAX 954.920.3729
www.yorkallergyusa.com

In addition to the organizations listed on the previous pages, these resources provide additional information and discussions on important topics:

www.enabling.org/ia/celiac (celiac disease, gluten sensitivities)
www.angelfire.com/mi/FAST (articles, recipes, and links)
www.foodprocessing.com (manufacturer links)
www.penny.ca/Links.htm (manufacturer links)
www.glutenfreeinfo.com/Diet/glutenfreeinfo.htm (manufacturer list)
www.celiac.com (celiac support page)
www.savorypalate.com (free recipes for gluten sensitivities)
www.allergykids.org/ (allergic kids' homepage)
www.funrsc.fairfield.edu/~jfleitas/kidsintro.html ("bandaids and blackboards")
POFAK-subscribe@yahoogroups.com (parents of allergic kids)
www.fankids.org (Food Allergy Network website for kids)
www.yeastconnection.com
www.allergybuyersclub.com (allergy resources, books, etc.)
www.nomilk.com (dairy sensitivities)

Mail-Order Sources

Wheat-Free/Gluten-Free Ingredients and Products

Authentic Foods
1850 W. 169 St., Suite B
Gardena, CA 90247
800.806.4737
FAX 310.366.7612
www.authenticfoods.com
Flours, ingredients, mixes

Better Batter
10835 Lawrence 1217
Mt. Vernon, MO 65712
417.466.DIET (3438)
www.betterbatter.com
Foods free of gluten and soy

Bob and Ruth's Travel Club
22 Breton Hill Rd., Suite 1B
Pikesville, MD 21208
410.486.0292
bobolevy@juno.com
Gluten-free newsletter and travel club

Bob's Red Mill Natural Foods
5209 S.E. International Way
Milwaukie, OR 97222
800.349.2173
FAX 503.653.1339
www.Bobsredmill.com
Flours, grains, mixes

Cybros, Inc.
417 Barney St.
Waukesha, WI 53186
800.876.2253
www.cybrosinc.com
Bakery items

Dietary Specialties
1248 Sussex Turnpike, Unit C-2
Randolph, NJ 07869
888.640.2800
www.dietspec.com
Foods, ingredients

Dowd and Rogers, Inc.
1641 49 St.
Sacramento, CA 95819
916.451.6480
FAX 916.736.2349
www.dowdandrogers.com
Chestnut flour mixes

Ener-G Foods, Inc.
5960 First Ave. S.
Seattle, WA 98124
800.331.5222
FAX 206.764.3398
www.ener-g.com
Flours, ingredients, mixes

Enjoy Life Foods
1601 Natchez Ave.
Chicago, IL 60707-4023
888.50.ENJOY
FAX 773.889.5090
www.enjoylifefoods.com
Cookies, bars, bagels

Gluten-Free Pantry
P.O. Box 840
Glastonbury, CT 06033
800.291.8386 (orders)
FAX 860.633.6853
www.glutenfree.com
Mixes, ingredients, appliances

Gluten Free Mall
www.glutenfreemall.com
Many vendors offering flours, ingredients, mixes, food, bakery items, books

Gluten-Free Market
1714 McHenry Rd.
Buffalo Grove, IL 60089
847.419.9610
FAX 847.419-9615
www.glutenfreemarket.com
Foods, ingredients, books

Gluten-Free Trading Co., LLC
604A W. Lincoln Ave.
Milwaukee, WI 53215
888.993.9933
FAX 414.385.9915
www.gluten-free.net
Flours, ingredients, mixes

Gluten Solutions, Inc.
3810 Riviera Dr., Suite 1
San Diego, CA 92109
888.845.8836
FAX 810.454.8277
www.glutensolutions.com
Mixes, ingredients, books, food

Glutino.com (DEROMA)
3750 Francis Hughes
Laval, Quebec, Canada H7L-5A9
800.363.DIET
FAX 450.629.4781
www.glutino.com
Mixes, ingredients, baked items

Goodday Health
514A N. Western Ave.
Lake Forest, IL 60045
877.395.2527
FAX 847.615.1209
gooddayglutenfree@msn.com
Gluten-free items, all major vendors

Jo's Spices Healthy Exchanges, Inc.
P.O. Box 124
DeWitt, IA 52742
563.659.8234
FAX 563.659.2126
www.healthyexchanges.com
Spice blends

King Arthur Flour
P.O. Box 876
Norwich, VT 05055-0876
800.827.6836
FAX 800.343-3002
www.bakerscatalogue.com
Flours, xanthan gum, mixes

Kinnikinnick Foods
10940-120 St.
Edmonton, AB, Canada, T5H 3P7
877.503.4466; 780.421.0456
www.kinnikinnick.com
Flours, foods, ingredients

Living Without (magazine)
P.O. Box 2126
Northbrook, IL 60065
847.480.8810
FAX 847.480.8819
www.livingwithout.com
Magazine for food sensitivities

Miss Roben's (Allergy Grocer)
91 Western Maryland Parkway, Suite 1
Hagerstown, MD 21740
800.891.0083
FAX 301.665.9584
www.missroben.com
Baking mixes, ingredients

Montina (Amazing Grains)
405 W. Main
Ronan, MT 59864
877.278.6585
FAX 406.676.0677
www.montina.com
Indian rice-grass flour, products

Nature's Hilights, Inc.
P.O. Box 3526
Chico, CA 95927
800.313.6454; 530.342.3130
www.natures-hilights.com
Pizza crusts, snacks, brownies

Pamela's Products
200 Clara Ave.
Ukiah, CA 95482
707.462.6605
FAX 707.462.6642
www.pamelasproducts.com
Cookies, mixes available from
    gluten-free vendors

Savory Palate, Inc.
8174 S. Holly, #404
Centennial, CO 80122-4004
800.741.5418
www.carolfenster.com
carol@carolfenster.com
Gluten-free cookbooks

Sylvan Border Farm
P.O. Box 277
Willits, CA 95490-0277
800.297.5399
FAX 707.459.1834
www.sylvanborderfarm.com
Mixes

Southwestern Ingredients

Chile Shop
109 E. Water St.
Santa Fe, NM 87501
505.983.6080
FAX 505.984.0737

Twin Valley Mills, LLC
R.R. 1, Box 45
Ruskin, NE 68974
402.279.3965
www.twinvalleymills.com
Sorghum flour

Vance's Foods
P.O. Box 255734
Sacramento, CA 95865
800.497.4834
FAX 800.497.4329
www.vancesfoods.com
Gluten-free milk powder and liquid

Index

About the Author

What began as a solution to Carol Fenster's own wheat intolerance grew into an internationally recognized publishing house serving people with food allergies, celiac disease, and autism. Today, Carol has published six books and is actively involved in and recognized as a leader in the area of food sensitivities. Her books are recognized by the Gluten Intolerance Group of North America, Celiac Disease Foundation, and Celiac Sprue Association as important resources for those with celiac disease. Many autism organizations support her work.

She developed a gluten-free product line for a national company, and she consults with manufacturers and teaches cooking classes. She appears on *Food for Life,* an allergy-free cooking show on the Health Network.

Her articles, recipes, and reviews of her books appear in magazines such as *Woman's World, Taste for Life, Vegetarian Times, Veggie Life, Better Nutrition, Gluten-Free Living,* and *Living Without;* professional journals such as *Today's Dietitian;* and newsletters from organizations such as Food Allergy and Anaphylaxis Network (FAAN), Gluten Intolerance Group, and Celiac Disease Foundation. She is the former Associate Food Editor of the magazine *Living Without: A Lifestyle Guide for People with Food & Chemical Sensitivities.*

Her recipes also appear in numerous books, including those published by the American Dietetic Association. She is a member of the International Association of Culinary Professionals.

She has a home economics degree from the University of Nebraska. Her doctorate is in Organizational Sociology from the University of Denver, where she was also a faculty member.